Nutrition Matters for Practice Nurses

*A handbook of dietary advice
for use in the community*

Dr Anthony R Leeds and Dr Patricia A Judd

Department of Nutrition and Dietetics
King's College London (formerly Queen Elizabeth College)
Campden Hill Road
London W8 7AH

Miss Brynda K Lewis

Department of Clinical Health Studies
Cardiff Institute of Higher Education
(formerly South Glamorgan Institute of Higher Education
Colchester Avenue
Cardiff CF3 7XR

The Editors and Publishers are pleased to acknowledge the sponsorship of this book by Quaker Oats Limited.

Nutrition Matters for Practice Nurses

Anthony R Leeds, Patricia A Judd and Brynda K Lewis

John Libbey

LONDON · PARIS

British Library Cataloguing in Publication Data
Leeds, Anthony R.
  Nutrition matters for practice nurses.
  1. Man. Nutrition
  I. Title II. Judd, Patricia III. Lewis, Brynda
613.2

ISBN: 0 86196 282 6

Published by
John Libbey & Company Ltd
13 Smiths Yard, Summerley Street, London SW18 4HR, England
Tel: +44 (0)81 947 2777
John Libbey Eurotext Ltd, 6 rue Blanche, 92120 Montrouge, France.
John Libbey - C.I.C. s.r.l., via L. Spallanzani 11, 00161 Rome, Italy

FOREWORD

This book arises from an idea which developed in the early summer of 1989 when it became apparent that practice nurses would be expected to give quite detailed dietary advice to patients seen in general practice. Specialist advice on diet from dietitians would be needed in some, perhaps more difficult, cases but there was little guidance on when the patient should be referred for such advice. The new GP contract with its requirements for health screening and the provision of dietary advice, and the development of coronary risk factor screening (then developing in some health districts) further emphasised the need.

Many individuals have contributed to this work. A team of enthusiastic practice nurses working near Cardiff was consulted about the needs and problems relating to diet as seen by practice nurses. The requested content was then produced in draft form by senior consulting dietitians on the staff of Nutrition and Dietetic Consultants. The draft chapters and supporting material were then scrutinised by the practice nurses – suggestions for modifications, additions and subtractions were obtained at six round table discussions. The vast task of editing to take account of the many views and opinions was then undertaken by the editors.

This work is, however, not just a book but a practical tool designed to facilitate the achievement of change in the diet of patients. To facilitate determination of the "baseline" diet a simple record sheet has been produced – this has been validated in trials by patients in five separate practices, is reproduced as an appendix to this book and is available on request from The Quaker Oats Nutrition Centre. To reinforce the messages given at the consultation five patient information leaflets have been produced, have been approved at round table discussions, are reproduced in the appendices, and again are available from The Quaker Oats Nutrition Centre.

As in all clinical management, flow-charts can help standardise treatment and ensure a better outcome for more patients. There is, however, debate about thresholds for action and criteria for inclusion in different treatment groups. The thresholds given in the text and flow-charts in this book are based on management guidelines either published or shortly to be published – an effort has been made to ensure that thresholds are as near consistent with other guidelines as is possible. Our flow-charts are, however, only suggestions and I hope that before putting them into use the primary health care team will discuss details and choose thresholds which take account of local needs and availability of services.

A number of areas are not covered by this book, and many questions will arise during management of specific patients. Your local dietitians are your best source of help with dietary problems – get in touch with the nearest hospital dietitian. In many areas the community dietitian will already have advised GP practices and many have produced literature on healthy eating and other topics. In some areas there may also be a preference that all patients use the locally produced diet sheets. If you do not know your local dietitian why not establish a channel of communication now?

During the course of reading and using this book you may come across errors or may wish to suggest improvements – please write to any of the editors with your views.

While designed primarily for practice nurses it is hoped that all or some of the content will be of use to other community nursing staff, perhaps also to some general practitioners and maybe to medical students or recently qualified medical staff who have a career in general practice in mind. It is also hoped that dietitians will recognize that we are trying to improve the quality of referral to them, rather than transfer their highly specialised skills to another group of health care professionals (which would be neither desirable nor possible).

Penny Barnett, Anne Masters Thomas, Elizabeth Simpson, Jeanie Swinburne and Patricia Walker were members of the team of writers at Nutrition and Dietetic Consultants who prepared the original texts. Scrutiny was undertaken by Sally Besch, Beryl Goodall, Mary Jones, Maureen Lewis, Rita Richards and June Smail – all members of the South Glamorgan Practice Nurses Association. Clinical photography (of patients who kindly gave permission for their photographs to be printed) was undertaken by Mike Ethrington of the Central Middlesex Hospital, London, and artwork and additional photography were done by Rodney Brown and Alan Rowland of King's College London. Preparation of patient advice leaflets has also involved personnel from The Quaker Oats Nutrition Centre who have worked with enthusiasm on the project. A number of colleagues have kindly reviewed work at various stages. I am particularly grateful to Dr Ewart Jepson, formerly of the Central Middlesex Hospital, London, Professor Marion Korczowski, formerly of the School of Nursing, Georgetown University, Washington, DC, and Dr Anne Stephenson, of the Department of General Practice and Primary Care, King's College School of Medicine and Dentistry, London, for their views. Sister Jenny Wootton, senior nurse (diabetes) at the Central Middlesex Hospital reviewed the chapter on diabetes. John Libbey has accepted multiple changes of text over the last few months with equanimity. I and my fellow editors, Patricia Judd and Brynda Lewis are very grateful to all contributors for their hard work.

Finally this project could not have been completed without the support of Dr Gerry Jewell, Director of Research and Development, Quaker Oats Ltd. I am grateful to him for his unconditional support throughout the last year, from discussion of ideas at the beginning to enthusiastic reception of the final product at the present time.

Anthony R Leeds

King's College London
29th August 1990

Contents

INTRODUCTION

The Role of the Practice Nurse in Management of Diet in Preventive and Therapeutic Situations

Over the past decade or so the importance of primary health care in contributing to health promotion has increasingly been emphasized. The World Health Organization European office has set targets for lifestyle, but also targets for the involvement of primary health care in health promotion[1]. The United Kingdom government has responded by including a number of health promotion and disease prevention activities in the latest contract for NHS general practitioners[2]. In the United Kingdom there are about 30,000 general practitioners and 8,000 practice nurses. Roughly 95% of the British population is registered with a GP. About 65% of men and 76% of women visit the surgery at least once a year, the highest consultation rates being for manual workers. In the past patients have sometimes been offered opportunistic health advice during consultations about other matters.

The GP contract implemented in April 1990 offers several new opportunities for screening and advice. All newly registered patients must be offered a consultation which should include discussion of lifestyle, and practices are now encouraged to set up health promotion clinics for which remuneration is provided by the Family Health Service Authorities. Elderly patients over 75 years of age must be offered annual check ups.

A key element in counselling about lifestyle is nutritional advice. The importance of healthy eating has been underlined in numerous official reports, such as that by the National Advisory Committee on Nutrition Education (NACNE), and the various reports of the Committee on Medical Aspects of Food Policy (COMA), in particular their report on diet and cardiovascular disease[3]. Lifestyle advice is not just about giving straightforward advice to patients, one must also examine

9

the health environment in which the patient lives and consider the barriers that may exist which prevent or make it difficult for the individual to adopt new health habits. Anyone giving nutritional advice in primary health care must not only be conversant with the patients' attitude towards food determined by their upbringing and cultural background, but must be aware of the economic functioning of the family, the availability of different foodstuffs locally and of the pressures created by big-business food advertising.

The food industry, mindful of its commercial interests, has recently developed and promoted "healthy" foods. Undoubtedly the consumer is at risk of becoming confused by the multiplicity of choice and may fail to understand the conflicting claims. How is the consumer to judge whether he or she should be concentrating on polyunsaturated fats or eating daily breakfasts of oat bran cereal? What does the word "polyunsaturated" mean to the average consumer and how important is the label "low in cholesterol"? The consumer not only needs sound general information on diet from the media and health education authorities but, crucially, needs to be able to consult a knowledgeable source for further advice.

Primary health care practitioners and, in particular, practice nurses are in a key position to give advice about nutritional matters. Both doctors and nurses have the background knowledge of the disease processes which are triggered by inappropriate diet, from constipation and piles to heart disease and certain types of cancer. Their advice can carry conviction, but only if it is drawn from a background knowledge of both disease processes and basic nutritional principles.

Reedy[4] refers to the work of practice nurses as counsellors, listeners and advisers. He says:

> *"It is common experience of practice nurses that patients see them as being more accessible than the doctor and easier to communicate with. They build up an informal relationship with the nurse which tends to allow and encourage unscheduled consultations with her and, as the depth of this relationship increases with time and extends to include more and more patients, she is increasingly used as the point of first contact in the surgery."*

American studies have shown that nurse practitioners have excellent outcomes in helping people change their lifestyles. One study found that nurse practitioners were effective at helping people lose weight, keep appointments, and comply with recommendations[5]. A British study showed similar results[6] when a nurse cared for hypertensive people in three general practices. Professional dietitians may be concerned that practice nurses may not be able to offer skilled advice to their patients. A recent study[7] demonstrated that a nurse counsellor working in a general practice setting was able to generate a real change in dietary habits among patients seen for health checks. This was reflected in the drop in plasma lipid levels compared to a control group who did not receive dietary advice. This contribution to the prevention of coronary heart disease, perhaps the greatest preventive challenge for primary care, also requires reduction in smoking and control of high blood pressure as well as a progressive reduction of obesity. Data from community surveys in the UK show that around one-third of the adult population may have cholesterol levels greater than 6.5 mmol/l, warranting at least active intervention with dietary advice[8]. The Oxford Heart Disease and Stroke Prevention Project has shown that it is feasible for practice nurses both to monitor dietary practices and to give dietary advice[9].

For centuries appropriate nutrition for patients suffering from a wide range of illnesses has been recognized as an essential feature of medical and nursing care. Today, practice nurses have many opportunities to give basic nutritional advice. They are involved in primary prevention activities, such as health promotion clinics. Secondary prevention (detection of pre-symptomatic disease) involves screening clinics and case-findings. Nutritional advice must be available wherever cholesterol testing is carried out. Tertiary prevention involves the management of established disease so as to limit complications, and is perhaps an area which is more familiar to nurses.

Practice nurses are increasingly organizing regularly structured reviews of patients with chronic diseases, such as hypertension and diabetes. They are, therefore, involved more and more in the giving of dietary advice which is important in the first line management of many of these conditions. Since they are already providing such dietary advice, it is important that the messages which they are disseminating are accurate and consistent.

There is now much scientific evidence of the benefit of improving the Western diet. No one enjoys being ill or watching members of their family suffer from heart disease, cancer or diabetes, illnesses which we know may have been prevented. Today we can make at least some strides towards better health by eating more wisely, and encouraging our patients to do likewise.

If we are to realize the World Health Organization's "Health for All" objectives, practice nurses must be appropriately trained to prepare them for their developing role, particularly in preventive and anticipatory care. Patients will be expecting the practice nurse to have up-to-date knowledge on all aspects of dietary advice.

In the last decade there has been an increase in the number of community dietitians, but their numbers are far too small to cope with the demand for education from the public. Dietitians play a vital role in educating the health professionals and liaising closely with primary health care teams. Provision of support for practice nurses and GPs in the form of expert advice on dietary management would ensure that consistent appropriate advice was being given to the patient. The practice nurse must also be able to recognize the need for professional dietetic intervention and understand the content of, and reasons for, current nutritional advice. The more a nurse knows about nutrition, the more likely she is to be able to refer patients appropriately for specialist dietary advice. Practice nurses have an individual responsibility to maintain and improve their professional knowledge and experience. The Welsh National Board has produced a framework for continuing education, "The Development of Professional Practice". This is a modular scheme which will enable practice nurses to obtain a Certificate and eventually a Diploma in Professional Practice. One of these modules available for practice nurses and other nurses working in the community will be "Applied Nutrition in

Health Care". The English National Board is currently review-
ing practice nurse training.

I hope that nutritional matters will become a core subject in
both basic and continuing education for practice nurses, given
the importance of the key task – that of improving the nation's
diet and diminishing the toll of the many diseases which can
be prevented by better nutrition.

June Smail

Practice and Research Sister
University of Wales College of Medicine
Llanedeyrn Health Centre
Cardiff
Chairman of South Glamorgan Practice Nurses Association
May 1990

References

1. WHO (1985): Targets for Health for All. WHO Regional Office for
   Europe, Copenhagen.

2. Department of Health (1990): Terms of Service for Doctors in General
   Practice. DoH, London.

3. Report of the Committee on Medical Aspects of Food Policy (1984):
   Diet and Cardiovascular Disease. DHSS Report HMSO, London.

4. Reedy, B. L. (1972): The general practice nurse. Update 5, 75-78.

5. Watkins, L. and Wagner, E. (1982): Nurse practitioner and physician
   adherence to standing orders criteria for consultations as referral.
   American Journal of Public Health, 72, 22-29.

6. Kenkre, J., Drury, V. W. and Lancashire, R. J. (1985): Nurse management of hypertension clinics in general practice, assisted by
   computer. Family Practice, 2(1), 17-22.

7. Baron, J. A., Gleason, R., Crowe, B. and Mann, J. I. (1990): Prelimi-
   nary results of general practice based nutritional advice. Journal
   of the Royal College of General Practitioners, 40, 333, 137-141.

8. Health Promotion Authority for Wales (1990): Health in Wales 1990.
   HPAW, Cardiff.

9. Fullard, E. M., Fowler, G. H. and Gray, J. A. M. (1987): Promoting
   prevention in primary care: controlled trial of low technology, low
   cost approach. British Medical Journal, 294, 1080-1082

Chapter 1

A HEALTHY LIFESTYLE

The idea that the diets of many people in the UK are damaging their health has now become almost universally accepted by the health professions. Much of the research and publications have been related particularly to coronary heart disease, but other conditions such as hypertension and stroke, diseases of the digestive system such as colon cancer and diverticular disease, obesity and dental caries, and possibly other cancers are all related to the food we eat.

Diet is not the only factor – in many cases the person's whole lifestyle may be putting them at risk. If we take Coronary Heart Disease (CHD) as an example, then smoking and exercise habits, and exposure to stress are facets of the patient's lifestyle which all need discussion.

What is a healthy diet?

The current consensus is that most people eat too much fat (especially saturated fat), salt and simple carbohydrates (sugars), and too little starchy carbohydrate and dietary fibre, and that we should therefore reduce consumption of the first three and increase the others. The NACNE and COMA reports put specific figures on these recommendations as shown in Appendix 1, but the most important thing to remember is that we eat foods not nutrients and for many people telling them to reduce their saturated fat intake may mean very little. Information about which foods contain fat, which to reduce and what to eat instead is essential.

The guidelines below are intended for healthy adults who are not overweight. If on routine screening or health check your patient is found to have a condition such as hyperlipidaemia or hypertension or is overweight, then there are some special dietary considerations which are detailed in subsequent chapters. However, even in these conditions the basic guidelines for a healthy diet still apply – it will just be necessary to stress some things in more detail.

It is important that a person's diet should include all their requirements for essential nutrients, such as protein, certain "essential" fatty acids, and vitamins and minerals, as well as supply an appropriate amount of energy. However, it is impossible to predict an individual's requirement with any accuracy and we fall back on the argument that if a person's energy needs are supplied by a variety of foods chosen sensibly, all these requirements will be met.

The basic aims of a healthy diet are therefore:

- **To supply an appropriate amount of energy and essential nutrients.**
- **To obtain about 50% of the energy from starchy carbohydrate foods.**
- **To increase dietary fibre intake to 30 g per day.**
- **To reduce fat intake to less than 35% of the energy intake.**
- **To reduce salt intake if excessive.**
- **To reduce sugar intake if this is high.**

What does your patient eat?

Before you start giving advice to anyone, you really need to have some idea of what they are eating at the moment. You can then target the advice to particular problem areas; many people will already have made some changes to their diet as a result of media or other information and your contribution will be better received if it takes into account the fact that they have already altered their diet.

You can do this by questioning the patient about particular foods or you could ask them to keep a record of what they eat for a few days and to bring it back for discussion. An example of a food record sheet which you could use is in Appendix F. Try to impress on the patient the importance of recording their normal diet, not changing what they eat while they are writing it down. Look at the record critically with respect to areas which might need attention and, if it seems helpful, "correct" the diet record by suggesting healthier options.

Changing food habits

It is often easier for people to make gradual changes to their eating habits rather than try to reform completely all at once. Some people may not be able to make the jump from poor choices of food to the best choices immediately, but can be persuaded to make smaller changes. A good example is trying to encourage someone to change to low fat milk – few people used to the taste and texture of whole milk take readily to skimmed milk, but many will try semi-skimmed as an interim measure and may be prepared to move on to skimmed milk later.

It is important to remember that you are trying to help people to make permanent changes in their lives and it may need to be a gradual process rather than a sudden "all or nothing" change.

The following sections deal with areas which may need attention in achieving the aims of a healthy diet and point out the things to look for when assessing your patient's diet, together with suggestions for change.

Energy and nutrient requirements

Energy

If an individual is at a sensible weight for his height (see Fig. 1 in Chapter 2) and stays within a kilogram or two of that weight, that individual has an appropriate energy intake for his current level of activity. If individuals increase their food intake or reduce their activity level (or perhaps more commonly, as they get older, decrease activity but maintain the same food intake), they will gain weight. Loss of weight will obviously occur if they reverse these processes. The range of energy intakes may be quite wide – a small sedentary woman may be eating as little as 1,200 Calories a day, whereas a young sportsman might need three times as much.

In each case the quality of the diet is important, ie what sorts of food are eaten and where the energy comes from. Ideally, the person should obtain more of their energy from starchy carbohydrate than fat and sugar, but in each case there may be problems. For the young woman it may be difficult to ensure that the diet is adequate in nutrients such as iron, and for the man, because a high energy, high starch diet is bulky, it may prove difficult for him to maintain his intake without resorting to sweet or fatty foods.

The energy in the diet is supplied by fat, carbohydrate (such as starches and sugars), protein, and alcohol. Fat is the most concentrated form of energy – every gram eaten supplies 9 Calories compared to around 4 Calories for protein and carbohydrate, and 7 from alcohol. This means that reducing fat intake is a very good way of cutting energy intake.

Essential nutrients

Certain nutrients are needed daily. With few exceptions, most people in this country obtain enough of all these nutrients and nutrient deficiency diseases are rare. The essential nutrients are proteins, essential fatty acids, vitamins and trace elements. Proteins are found in concentrated amounts in meat, fish, egg, milk, cheese and pulses and are important constituents of cereals. Provided that the following basic dietary habits are observed, protein intake will take care of itself. This also applies to the essential fatty acids which are supplied in sufficient amounts by all normal diets. As far as vitamins and minerals are concerned, it is possible sometimes to have low intakes of these, but again the guidelines below should ensure that all requirements are covered. There are tables giving more information on vitamins and minerals in Chapter 8.

Fat

Fats are composed of basic units, fatty acids, of which about 21 are important in the diet. According to their chemical makeup, these can be described as saturated (SFA) or unsaturated – the former are usually hard at room temperature and the latter oils. Food fats contain a mixture of fatty acids and no fat is completely saturated or unsaturated. Saturated fats raise blood cholesterol levels, polyunsaturated fats (PUFA) lower them and recent research suggests that monounsaturated fats (MUFA), such as those found in olive or rapeseed oils, may be useful in the diet because they don't raise cholesterol levels and don't have some of the possible disadvantages of high intakes of PUFA.

Foods containing mostly saturated fatty acids are:

■ **Butter, lard, hard margarine, fatty meats and meat products such as sausages and patés.**

Foods containing mostly monounsaturated fatty acids are:

■ **Olive, rapeseed and groundnut oils.**

Foods containing mostly polyunsaturated fatty acids are:

■ **Corn, sunflower, soya, safflower oils and margarines made from them.**

On average, just over 42% of the energy in the UK diet comes from fat, of which half is saturated fat. It is now considered important to reduce the amount of energy from fat to about one-third of the energy in the diet and that only 10% should come from saturated fats.

Table 1 shows which foods are high in fat and how to replace these with less fatty substitutes.

Many of the people you advise to reduce fat intake are likely to be overweight and will therefore benefit from the concomitant fall in energy intake. However there will be some people with an undesirably high fat intake who are not overweight, but who are likely to lose weight unless they are given specific advice. For these people, it is even more important to stress the switch to high carbohydrate foods as discussed below.

Table 1. Foods with high, medium and low fat content

HIGH	MEDIUM	LOW
Whole milk	Semi-skimmed milk	Skimmed milk
Cheeses - most hard, eg cheddar, cream cheese	Edam, brie, camembert, low-fat hard cheeses, eg Shape, Tendale	Cottage cheese, low fat curd cheeses, fromage frais
Fatty meat, meat products, eg sausages, bacon, pasties, pies	Red meat - beef, pork, lamb	Poultry - chicken, turkey
Mackerel, herring*	Salmon, trout, tuna	White fish - cod, plaice, haddock, whiting
Cakes, pastries, sweets, chocolate biscuits	Scones, plain biscuits, cream crackers	Crispbreads, teacakes, plain yeast bun
Butter, margarines	Low fat spreads	
Mayonnaise, salad cream	Low fat versions of salad cream and mayonnaise	Low fat dressings

General note: Encourage patients to grill, bake, boil or steam foods rather than fry.

* Fatty fish once or twice a week may be good as fatty fish is high in PUFA and its use can be encouraged unless the patient is overweight.

You may be asked about some specific fatty acids which are being talked about in the media now because they seem to have some beneficial effects.

Linoleic acid is a polyunsaturated fatty acid which we must obtain from our food because we cannot make it ourselves – hence it is an essential fatty acid. Fortunately, we need only a small amount each day and, provided some fat is eaten, we do not become deficient. A fatty acid with a somewhat similar name is gamma-linolenic acid (GLA), which is made in the body in small amounts from linoleic acid. Evening primrose oil (EPO) is a rich source of GLA and is sold as a dietary supplement. Many claims have been made for EPO, eg that it relieves the symptoms of premenstrual tension, but its role in the treatment of eczema has been established. It has also been suggested to help in multiple sclerosis in conjunction with a low fat diet.

Fish oils contain specific PUFA which may have useful effects. The oils which come from the body of the fish (and which can, therefore, be obtained by eating fatty fish such as mackerel) seem to help prevent blood clotting and therefore help prevent CHD. This oil can also be taken in concentrated form as a supplement by those who don't like fish, but supplements are expensive. Cod liver oil may also have beneficial effects – it has been suggested that it may help people with psoriasis and some other skin diseases and, of course, it is high in vitamins A and D.

Increasing starchy carbohydrates

In the past, bread, potatoes, cereals and starchy foods generally used to be regarded as bad for you. Some people blame their spreading waistlines on these sorts of foods, but if you think about it carefully, it is often not these foods alone which are to blame but a combination of starch with fat and sugar in puddings, cakes or biscuits which increase the energy content markedly. We now believe that it is best to base our diet on starchy staple foods, such as bread, pasta, rice or other whole grains and starchy roots like potato. It has been suggested that instead of thinking of meals as, for example, meat and potato and vegetables it would be a good idea to reverse this and think along the line of potatoes, vegetables and ... . This puts the staple food first and the meat or cheese or other high protein food into a more appropriate position and may also help to get across the idea that a small amount of it is all that is needed at each meal. In fact, all these staple foods contain some protein and adding a small amount of animal protein or indeed more vegetable protein such as beans or pulses is all that is needed to balance the diet.

Vegetables and fruit also contain carbohydrate in various forms and are recommended as part of a healthy diet. On the whole they are low in energy and supply many useful vitamins and minerals as well as some dietary fibre.

Because the carbohydrate in these recommended foods is intimately mixed with the dietary fibre, it is digested and absorbed slowly and metabolism is controlled, with beneficial effects on blood sugar levels.

Carbohydrates supply only 4 Calories for every gram eaten compared to the 9 supplied per gram of fat, so if the person is to maintain the same energy intake when they reduce their fat intake they will need to eat, weight for weight, more of the starchy foods. This is sometimes a problem, especially for people who have high energy requirements. They will need encouragement to eat more bread and bigger portions of potatoes, rice, pasta, without the butter or oil which they may be used to adding. Suggestions such as cutting bread more thickly and using soft margarine to spread thinly or using plain yoghurt as a dressing for potato rather than butter or mayonnaise may help. Of course this bulking effect is useful if people need to lose weight – encouraging them to continue with the same intake of starchy foods but cut the fat works wonders.

Restricting sugar intake

Sugars are also carbohydrates – there are many different kinds of sugars in the diet, but those we eat most of are sucrose, otherwise known simply as sugar, and lactose, the sugar in milk. A recent government report concluded that sugar *per se* was not implicated in disorders such as obesity and heart disease, though it was agreed that dental caries was related to sugar consumption. However, it has been suggested by other committees that the sugar intake in this country should not increase. There are many foods, like cakes, biscuits, and confectionery, which are highly palatable and energy-rich and simply would not be eaten if sugar did not exist. Few people would eat cocoa and cocoa butter alone, but add sugar and the resulting chocolate is irresistible to many.

If your patient is overweight and takes sugar in drinks or drinks sugary squashes or fizzy drinks, then suggest that they stop taking sugar (or use an artificial sweetener if they must) and change to low calorie soft drinks. This removes nothing from the diet but the energy as sugar contains no other nutrients. Sweets and chocolates are best replaced with fruit.

Increasing dietary fibre

Dietary fibre is also largely carbohydrate but differs from those mentioned above because we are not able to digest it and absorb the sugars which it contains. It used to be thought that dietary fibre was inert and simply passed through the gut unchanged and that its only beneficial effect was to prevent constipation. We now understand more about this complex dietary constituent and believe that it has important effects both in the bowel and in other parts of the body. A high fibre intake protects against constipation and may also prevent some of the disorders that accompany constipation, such as diverticulitis and haemorrhoids. Some research has suggested that a high fibre intake is protective against colon cancer, though this is difficult to prove. Evidence also suggests that certain types of fibre, the so-called soluble fibre found especially in foods like oat bran and leguminous seeds, modify the way nutrients are absorbed in the gut and may, therefore, reduce blood cholesterol levels. A high fibre diet is a bulky diet and helps to prevent patients feeling hungry when eating a diet low in fat and sugar.

How to do it

By encouraging your patients to eat more starchy carbohydrate foods and vegetables and fruit, you will automatically be encouraging them to eat more fibre, but some extra advice may be needed. Appendix 2 below shows sources of dietary fibre in the diet.

Again people may find it difficult to change from a low fibre diet to a high fibre diet overnight. If they make gradual changes, it is possible that they will suffer fewer of the side effects which sometimes put people off, ie feeling bloated and uncomfortable and producing more wind than usual.

Some practical ideas for increasing fibre:

■ **Change to wholemeal bread. (But remember white bread does contain fibre and if someone doesn't like wholemeal bread, it's better to eat white than none at all - suggest they increase the amount of bread generally).**

■ **Eat a wholegrain cereal rather than a refined one - eg Shredded Wheat rather than cornflakes. Porridge is a good high fibre breakfast dish, containing soluble fibre, which may help to lower blood cholesterol. Oat bran and oat bran products contain larger amounts of soluble fibre.**

■ **Replace some of the flour in all baked goods with wholemeal flour - gradually increase the amount as people get used to it.**

■ **Replace some of the meat in stews and other dishes with beans - eg chilli con carne with red kidney beans, tuna fish with butter beans in a salad. Gradually reduce the meat or fish and increase the beans.**

It is important for people to have an adequate fluid intake on a high fibre diet, so encourage your patients to drink at least three pints of liquids per day.

It has been suggested that the ideal intake of dietary fibre for an adult is between 30–35 g per day, but there is no need for people to add up every gram – if they are passing one or two soft stools each day without straining, they are probably eating enough fibre.

Reducing salt intake

Most people in this country take much more salt in the diet than they really need. As well as the salt added to food at the table and in cooking, many processed foods contain large amounts of salt. Cheeses, bacon, ham and other cured meats, smoked meats and fish, canned meats and vegetables, canned and packet soups, sauces and pickles all contain hidden salt.

There is some controversy as to whether everybody in the country should be encouraged to cut down on salt since it has been suggested that only between 10–20% of the population are susceptible to high salt intakes in the sense of developing hypertension. However, cutting down on salt is unlikely to do any harm and may be beneficial, so it is worth asking your patient a few questions about salt intake and giving some advice. Ask the patient about salt added to food and in cooking and if they use a lot, advise them to cut down. If they eat processed foods regularly, such as canned meats, soups and vegetables, then encourage them to change to fresh versions. More detailed information on this topic is given in the chapter on hypertension as, if the patient is found to be hypertensive, salt reduction has definite benefits.

Alcohol intake

Alcohol supplies calories (7 per g) and therefore should be strictly limited by those trying to lose weight. It is harmful in even relatively small amounts depending partly on the person's sex and weight. The recommended maximum is 3 standard drinks per day for men and 2 for women.

A standard drink is equivalent to:

- ½ pint of beer, cider or lager
- 1 measure of spirits
- 1 small glass of wine or sherry

If your patient is trying to lose weight it is best to encourage them to strictly limit alcohol consumption – in many cases all good intentions about eating less are rapidly forgotten after a few drinks.

Changing food habits

Table 2 shows a typical day's diet and the changes which could be advised to improve it. As the fat intake goes down from left to right, the patient who is not overweight should increase the amounts of bread and potatoes, and eat extra fruit if hungry.

Table 2. A typical day's diet and suggested changes

	Poor	Better	Best
Breakfast	Fried egg, fried bacon, fried white bread, white toast, butter, marmalade. Tea, whole milk, sugar.	Poached egg on wholemeal toast, butter, marmalade. Tea, semi-skimmed milk sweetener.	High fibre cereal, wholemeal toast, PUFA margarine, marmalade. Skim milk on cereal and in tea.
Mid-morning	Coffee, milk, sugar, chocolate shortbread.	Coffee, semi-skimmed milk, digestive biscuit.	Coffee, skimmed-milk, apple.
Lunch	Sandwiches, white bread, butter, tuna mayonnaise, doughnut, coca-cola.	Sandwiches, brown bread, PUFA margarine, tuna mayonnaise, iced bun, diet coke.	Sandwiches, whole meal bread, PUFA margarine, tuna and salad, fruit, fruit juice/water.
Tea	Cream cake. Tea, milk, sugar.	Fruit cake. Tea, semi-skimmed milk.	Scone and PUFA margarine. Tea, skimmed-milk.
Supper	Steak pie, mashed potatoes with butter & milk, carrots, sponge pudding and custard.	Beef stew, mashed potatoes and PUFA, carrots, stewed fruit and semi-skimmed custard.	Beef and bean stew, baked potato, carrots, stewed fruit and low fat yoghurt.
Bedtime	Drinking chocolate with whole milk, 3 cream crackers, cheese & butter.	Drinking chocolate with semi-skimmed milk, 2 cream crackers, low fat cheese.	Malted milk with skimmed milk, 2 crisp breads, low fat cheese spread.

Other aspects of a healthy lifestyle

Diet is not the only factor which needs to be considered in achieving a healthy lifestyle – other factors such as exercise and smoking habits and exposure to stress are also important.

Detailed consideration of these is not within the scope of this book but a few comments are necessary.

Smoking

Cigarette smoking is probably the most unhealthy habit anyone can have and should be discouraged as much as possible. It is especially important to try to help the patient to stop smoking if they are hypertensive, have diabetes or hyper-lipidaemia or signs of CHD. There are leaflets available to general practices which you may find helpful to give to the patient.

Exercise

Exercise should be encouraged as part of the daily life of all your patients. Many will be very inactive and should be encouraged to include some form of exercise into their daily life This does not mean persuading the inactive person to start jogging three times each week – gentle exercise which can be incorporated into day-to-day activity is all that is required to start. Walking for 15 to 20 minutes each day, climbing stairs instead of taking the lift, or taking the dog out for a walk are all exercise. Swimming can be good exercise for those who have joint problems as the water supports the weight.

If you have any doubt about the advisabilty of encouraging a patient to take exercise consult the doctor. If they have not exercised for some time or are unfit, stress the need to start with gentle exercise and build it up gradually.

Stress

Modern life puts people into many stressful situations and this can exacerbate problems such as high blood pressure, hyper-lipidaemia and even obesity if the person overeats in response to the stress. Exercise can be an antidote to stress and there are also many relaxation techniques which can be used to alleviate it. It may be worth finding out about what is available in your area so that you can direct patients who need help towards sensible advice.

Special groups

Children

The changes in the diet advocated now are intended to help prevent diseases which show themselves in later life, but may already be developing in childhood. In older children, the sort of dietary changes advocated above are unlikely to do any harm, but in pre-school children should not be taken to extremes. Children have higher nutrient requirements weight for weight than adults because not only do they have to replace tissues, but they are growing as well. The energy needs of a five-year old may be as high as those of an adult, but the child will have a smaller capacity for food and giving a very low fat diet, high in starchy carbohydrate and fibre may prove so bulky that the child simply cannot eat enough to get the energy he needs.

For these reasons it is advocated that children under two are given whole milk rather than low fat versions. Between two and five this can be changed to semi-skimmed milk, provided the child eats a variety of other foods supplying energy. Wholegrain cereals and bread can be given, but if the child has a small appetite it may be better not to give bulky meals based on cereals and pulses but to ensure energy and iron intakes by giving meat and fish daily.

Children are the one group who can be seen to benefit most from limiting sugar intake – in terms of preventing tooth decay. It has been shown that the number of occasions in a day that sugar is taken is crucial. It may not be possible to ban sweets completely, but suggest that they are given at the end of a meal rather than between meals and not too frequently.

Pregnancy

During pregnancy it is important for the health of the mother and child that a healthy diet is taken. Pregnant women are often very receptive to advice about diet because they are keen to do their best for their baby. The diet should be based on the principles above, but some nutrients need special care. When checking the diet look especially carefully for foods which supply calcium, eg milk, cheese, yoghurt. A pregnant woman needs more calcium than normal and should be advised to make sure she has the equivalent of a pint of milk each day as either low fat milk or yoghurt. Low fat cheeses can be used, but cottage cheese is not as rich in calcium as the hard version. Many antenatal clinics now suggest that fermented soft cheeses as well as paté are to be avoided during pregnancy because of the danger of infection with *Listeria sp.* For this reason also, pregnant women are advised to cook well all meats and made-up dishes.

Adequate iron intake is also important in pregnancy and the woman should be encouraged to have some red meat at least 3–4 times per week, cutting off all the fat. Liver once each week if the woman likes it will ensure an adequate intake. Iron is present in vegetable foods like cereals and pulse vegetables, but is less well absorbed than from meat. Vitamin C aids absorption so a glass of orange juice or a salad with meals can help.

The high fibre diet with plenty of fluids advocated above will help prevent the constipation which is common in pregnancy, but as the baby grows and takes up more space it may become difficult to eat bulky meals. Small meals and snacks may be the answer here.

Ethnic minority groups

It is important to take into account a person's culture and food habits when advising about diet. Many minority groups have rules about eating laid down as part of their religion and will not take your advice if it goes against this, so if any of your patients are of a different race or creed it is worth finding out more about their specific food rules. Appendix 3 outlines the basics of the rules about diet of the major religions, but if you see many such patients in your practice, contact your local dietitians as it is likely that they will have prepared special information sheets for the different ethnic groups which they may wish you to use.

Vegetarians

Many vegetarians are very health conscious and will be well aware of what consitutes a healthy diet. However, a lacto-ovo vegetarian diet, in which a lot of dairy produce and eggs is eaten, is not necessarily lower in fat than an omnivorous diet. These people may, therefore, benefit from using low fat dairy products. In the vegan diet no animal products are eaten and this can be a very healthy diet as long as mixtures of cereal beans and nuts are eaten to give an adequate protein intake. Most vegans are aware that their diet can be lacking in vitamin B12, but those new to the regimen should be advised to take some yeast extract each day to provide the vitamin.

The problem vegetarian is typically a teenager who decides to stop eating animal products, but does not think about how to replace the nutrients he/she was previously getting from these foods. They should be advised to eat mixtures of cereals and beans or nuts as well as vegetables, if they do not intend to eat dairy products, and have a source of vitamin B12.

Chapter 2

OBESITY

1.What is it?

When the intake of energy from the diet exceeds the output of energy then the excess is stored as adipose tissue, mainly under the skin. As the layer of adipose tissue becomes thicker, body weight rises. Once body weight exceeds that which is recommended for a person's age, sex and height then that person may be classed as overweight or obese, depending upon their actual body weight.

In practice, the best method of assessing by how much a particular person is overweight is to calculate their body mass index (BMI):

$$BMI = \frac{Weight \ (kg)}{Height \ (m^2)}$$

Height is taken without shoes and weight without shoes and in indoor clothing.

The number produced by the calculation of BMI can then be used to help classify obesity, as indicated in Table 1.

Table 1. Classification of obesity using BMI

BMI:	CLASSIFICATION:
< 20	Underweight
20 - 24.9	Grade 0 - normal
25 - 29.9	Grade 1 - overweight
30 - 40	Grade 2 - obesity
> 40	Grade 3 - severe obesity

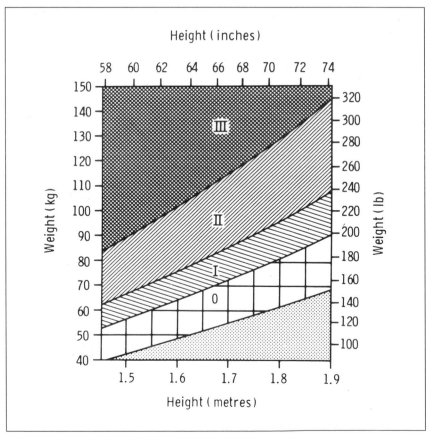

Fig. 1. Height and weight related. (Reproduced with permission from J S Garrow: Treat obesity seriously: Churchill Livingstone, Edinburgh 1981)

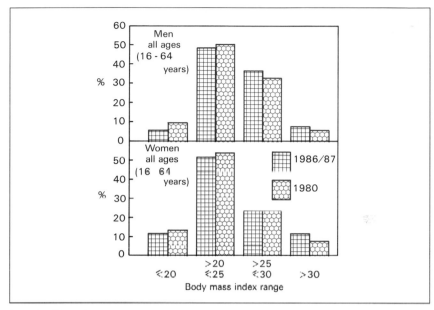

Fig. 2. Distribution (as a percentage) of men and women (aged 16-64 years) in body mass index groups in 1980 (The heights and weights of adults in Great Britain, Ian Knight, OPCS, HMSO, 1984) and 1986/87 (The dietary and nutritional survey of British adults, Janet Gregory et al, OPCS, HMSO, 1990).

Fig. 3. Changes (as a percentage) of distribution of men and women (aged 16-64 years) in body mass index groups between 1980 and 1986/87 - sources described in the legend to Fig. 2.

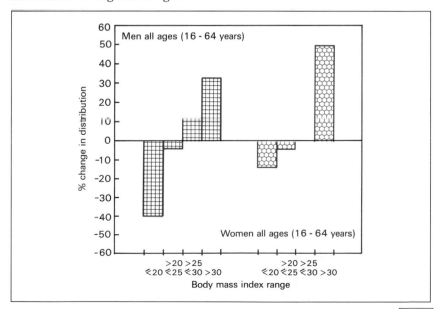

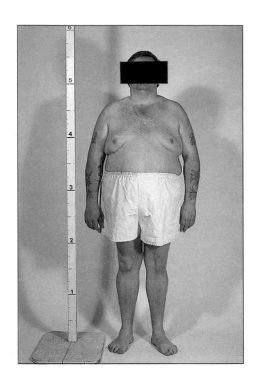
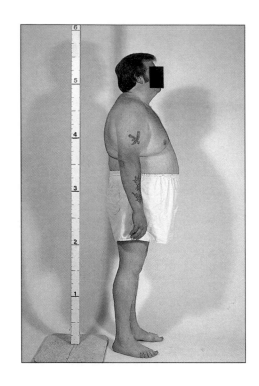
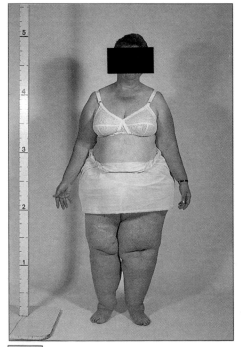
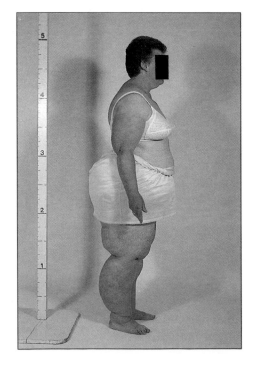

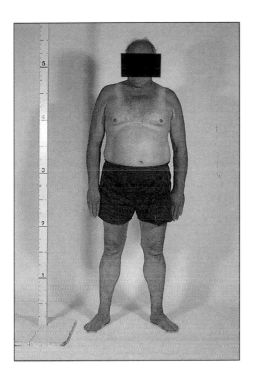 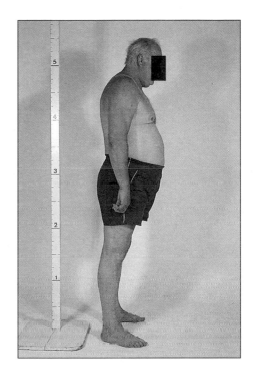

Fig. 4. (facing page, top). A patient with centrally distributed adipose tissue: Body Mass Index 41.2 (Weight 122 kg, Height 172 cm), waist/hip ratio 1.13 (Waist 137 cm, Hip 121 cm). The threshold value for waist/hip ratio in men is 1.0 – above this value the risk of metabolic disease is high. The patient has diabetes mellitus.

Fig. 5. (facing page, bottom). A patient with peripherally distributed adipose tissue: Body Mass Index 44.9 (Weight 115 kg, Height 160 cm), waist/hip ratio 0.66 (Waist 102 cm, Hip 154 cm). The threshold value for waist/hip ratio in women is 0.8 – above this value the risk of metabolic disease is high. This patient has no metabolic disease.

Fig. 6. (this page). A patient with centrally distributed adipose tissue: Body Mass Index 32.4 (Weight 97 kg, Height 173 cm), waist/hip ratio 1.02 (Waist 110 cm, Hip 108 cm). This patient has a hyperlipidaemia

It is important to remember that the classification is somewhat arbitrary and that, especially when a person is at the borderline for a grade, it will be necessary to consider carefully the treatment required. Confirmation of the degree of obesity may be obtained by plotting the person's height and weight on Fig. 1.

There is now evidence that the distribution of fat relates to risk of metabolic disease (CHD, diabetes and hyperlipidaemia). Central obesity where fat occurs in and around the abdomen increases the risk of such disease, whereas peripherally distributed fat does not. Measurement of the waist/hip ratio to assess this risk may become a common practice in future (see Figs. 4–6).

2. Is it a problem?

Obesity has been called the malnutrition of the affluent, but not all the affluent are obese and there are more obese people among the lower social classes.

There are more obese people in middle-aged and "young" elderly groups than in younger age groups, and more people are obese now than eight to ten years ago (see Fig. 2). The increase in the numbers of obese people (and the decrease in numbers of slim people) is shown graphically in Fig. 3. The amount of change (a 50% increase in the number of women with a BMI over 30 over a period of just seven years) is quite alarming.

To suggest that obesity is caused simply by eating too much is to understate the problem. In any one person there will be a number of psychological and social factors interacting to produce abnormal eating behaviour. It is beyond the scope of this book to pursue these factors in any detail, but the reading list contains some useful references (see Appendix 5).

As well as a psychological cause, obesity may have a profound psychological effect. The obese person may find themselves in a viscious circle where, being depressed because of their weight, they eat for comfort, thus putting on more weight. Breaking the circle is difficult, as is finding a substitute for food as a comforter.

To be obese is not socially acceptable in our society. Finding fashionable clothes is difficult, seats on public transport may not always be wide enough, and the obese are often ridiculed. Because of their size, many obese people are not very active and do not take part in sport. All of these factors will contribute to both obesity and the maintenance of a heavy body weight.

Obesity may also result in, or contribute to, a number of disorders which will then have an affect on health. The joints may be affected particularly by having to carry a heavy body weight so the person may be more prone to arthritis, especially of the weight-bearing joints – hips and knees. Non-insulin dependent diabetes is much more common in obese people, and the obese are more prone to varicose veins and hypertension. Obesity is also a recognized risk factor for coronary heart disease, the more severe the obesity the greater the risk. When obesity is severe, then life expectancy is reduced. Thus it is important that some attempt is made to reduce a heavy body weight for the future well-being of the patient.

3. How best might it be treated?

The treatment of obesity is individual; what suits one person will not necessarily suit all. Treatment may be best classified as either dietary or non-dietary, although it must be remembered that the majority of non-dietary treatments will require some modification of diet. A flow chart for the treatment of obesity is given in Fig. 7.

(1) Dietary treatment

(a) Healthy eating

Any good weight reducing diet should teach the principles of healthy eating outlined in Chapter 1. A healthy diet of a lower energy value than the patient's normal diet will provide a firm basis for weight loss and, importantly, maintenance of that loss. Successful weight loss can be achieved only if the patient is motivated to change his/her eating habits and to adopt a more healthy lifestyle; it is impossible to achieve if the patient does not want to lose weight.

In order to begin education on new eating habits, one must be aware of old habits. The best way of learning about a patient's food habits is to ask them to keep a diet diary for one week before they have any nutritional advice. It is important that the diary should be as honest a record as possible and that the patient does not change their eating habits during that week. This diary then becomes the patient's diet history and should be used as a basis for discussion of the good and bad points of the patient's current diet. The diary should also form the basis for discussion of the new eating habits so that changes can be agreed with the patient rather than being forced upon them.

The most important foods to look for are those which contain either a lot of fat or a lot of sugar, or both. The majority of these foods can then be replaced by lower fat or lower sugar alternatives or, if this is impossible, can be removed from the diet on a temporary basis. Patients should be encouraged to try to give up sugar in drinks preferably completely, although a non-nutritive sweetener may be used if necessary (see Table 2). Fizzy drinks and squashes should be of the "diet" variety and all forms of sweets, chocolates, cakes and pastries should be discouraged other than as a treat (see later).

The most obvious fats are the spreading and cooking fats and low fat spreads are a very suitable substitute. Patients should be discouraged from frying foods or keep them to a minimum and use a non-stick pan if possible. Most foods which are fried can be grilled and a microwave is very useful for low fat cooking if there is one available. Full fat milk can be changed to semi-skimmed or skimmed, and full fat cheeses to lower fat varieties. Meats should be as lean as possible, or affordable, and fish should be encouraged. Where meat products, such as sausages or beefburgers, feature in the diet, a low fat variety should be suggested.

Having looked at fat and sugar sources, fibre comes next. This means suggesting wholemeal or other high fibre breads, cereals and pastas, plus an increase in fruit and vegetable intake where possible. The healthy eating plan which explains all these changes in greater detail is given in Chapter 1. As part of the healthy eating plan, regular meals should be encouraged.

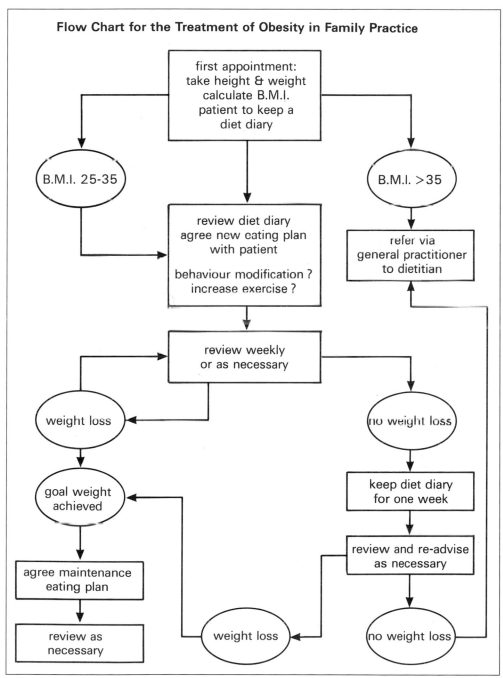

Flow Chart for the Treatment of Obesity in Family Practice

Fig. 7. Flow chart for the treatment of obesity in family practice. This sequence represents just one possible layout - in your own practice you may choose different thresholds and time intervals.

Patients should be discouraged from missing meals as a means of speeding up weight loss because, apart from not producing a nutritionally sound diet, it rarely works. Once people begin eating, they will find it difficult to stop and can consume more energy in a few short hours during the evening than during a whole day of well balanced, healthy meals.

As well as eating, patients must be encouraged to drink plenty, especially if they are changing to a high fibre intake. At least 3 pints of fluid each day should be recommended to avoid dehydration and the consequent evening headaches.

These small changes will cause a reduction in energy intake enough to start a loss in weight which may be sustained over a number of weeks or months.

Table 2. Suitable non-nutritive sweeteners	
Saccharin	All found in a variety of branded
Aspartame	sweeteners, such as Hermesetas, Sweetex,
Acesulfame-K	Flix, and Canderel

(b) Counting calories

This method of dieting to lose weight is very popular, mainly because it gives people control over their eating and the amount of energy they choose to consume each day. The main disadvantage is that it is easy to become calorie-orientated rather than food-orientated, so that good nutrition does not play any part in the diet – for example, a day's calorie allowance may be made up from bread, biscuits, beer and chocolate. However, it does teach people about the energy value of food and, providing they are also taught how to use a calorie chart properly, can be a useful means of dieting to lose weight for those who are interested in this method. A calorie chart is included as Appendix 4.

(c) Unusual diets

It is beyond the scope of this book to go into any great detail about the myriad of diets now available which purport to help people lose weight. Many are not nutritionally sound and do not promote long-term sensible eating habits. If you are asked about such a diet, then compare it with the guidelines for healthy eating given in Chapter 1 and Appendix 1. If the diet is a long way from these principles, then it is best to discourage its use.

However, it is worth looking in a little detail at the very low calorie liquid diets (VLCDs) which are now available. These diets can be bought from a chemist, health food shop, or from a company representative, known as a nutrition counsellor, who will sell the product direct, often to the person in their own home. The VLCD becomes the sole source of nutrition for some three to four weeks, after which time one meal each day for one week should be replaced by "normal" food. The VLCD can then become the sole source of nutrition for a further three weeks, and the cycle can be repeated until the required weight loss is achieved. The majority of companies who produce these diets also include a leaflet containing suggestions for meals, or produce their own meal-substitutes for patients to buy. They also offer advice on maintenance once weight is lost. VLCDs are popular because they offer quick weight loss without the bother of deciding which food to eat. The more reputable ones are nutritionally complete while containing only 600 Calories in one day's drinks. Unfortunately, the majority of people who use such diets put back all the weight they have lost and more once they stop the diet. The use of VLCDs as a means of weight loss has not had any long term success and the method does not teach the patient either good nutrition or sensible eating habits.

(d) Adjuncts to the diet

(i) Setting goals

Setting goals is an important part of the weight loss process, but the goals must be realistic, particularly where they relate to the amount of weight to be lost. It may not always be suitable

41

to calculate a person's ideal weight if they are three to four stones above it. A better ploy would be to set a target loss of one stone and then aim to review once that stone is lost. Realism also applies to goals such as giving up sugar or sweets. It is much better to agree to attempt one less spoonful of sugar in drinks this week and to carry on a gradual decrease over a month or so. This again helps the patient to feel in control of their food intake and weight loss.

(ii) Behaviour modification

A healthy eating plan should be combined with some simple behaviour modification techniques where appropriate. Behaviour modification teaches the patient to recognize, and so manipulate, those triggers which result in eating. Such triggers may be boredom, loneliness, sight or smell of food, mood change, or simply being in a room which is associated with food. A diary is a very useful tool in the identification of triggers and can be combined with a diet diary such that the patient is recording what they eat, why they are eating, how they feel before, during and after eating, and where they are at the time of eating. A behaviour/diet diary thus focusses the patient on to the reasons for their eating as well as the actual food which they consume. The diary can be used as a means of education and may be helpful to some patients as a way of monitoring their dieting behaviour.

Any or all of the techniques listed below will be useful adjuncts to the diet.

- **Plan your meals for the week if possible so that you do not have to shop on impulse.**
- **Never shop on an empty stomach.**
- **Make a shopping list and buy only the foods on the list.**
- **Take only enough money (if appropriate) to buy only the foods on the list.**
- **Cook only enough food for the numbers being served - no extra "for the pot" !**
- **Eat only in one room - ban eating from all other rooms.**
- **Keep food only in the kitchen - do not eat in the kitchen (unless it is the normal eating place in the house).**

■ **Do not do anything else while eating - no watching television, reading the paper or a book.**

■ **Eat from a smaller plate.**

■ **Put down your knife and fork in between mouthfuls.**

■ **Eat very slowly and chew well.**

■ **Try not to eat any food which does not require a knife and fork or spoon.**

(iii) "Legal cheating"

Most people will be unable to give up for all time those foods which they love, such as crisps, cakes or chocolate, therefore it is a good idea to build in these foods as part of the diet. They can be used within a reward system where, if the patient has rigidly kept to the agreed diet plan for seven days, on the eighth day they are allowed to "cheat" by eating a food which would normally be "forbidden". This allows the patient to choose their own treats and helps to teach them how to use such foods as part of a balanced eating plan. It also acts as a motivator! However, it is not essential and, if a patient decides that cheating is not for them on the basis that if they taste a small amount of their favourite food then they will find it very difficult to stop, then do not encourage cheating.

(iv) Exercise

Wherever possible it is also a good idea to suggest an increase in energy output. This may mean encouraging the patient to walk more or to try a sport, such as swimming. Increasing exercise has a two-fold advantage: it increases basal metabolic rate and so will help weight loss and a feeling of well-being, and it occupies the person, preventing boredom and a consequent increase in food intake.

(v) Support

As important as all the diet and lifestyle advice is the support that the practice nurse can give while the patient is trying to lose weight. For many people, the support is more important than the actual advice for they are aware of their bad eating habits and how they should be changed. The patient should be seen as regularly as they require and as time will allow. At each visit, the patient should be weighed and congratulated on any weight loss. If there is no weight loss, then a review of the diet should be undertaken to ensure that the patient is not eating too much. It may also be useful to ask the patient to keep another diet diary for one week. If the practice nurse is unable to ascertain the reason for no weight loss, then the patient should be referred, via the GP, to the dietitian.

(2) Non-dietary treatment

(a) Drugs

A large number of obese people visit their general practitioners to request a drug to help them lose weight, but few doctors prescribe such drugs. Although the drugs are effective at reducing appetite while they are being taken, once the patient stops the drug appetite returns and weight gain often occurs. Therefore, appetite reducing drugs are not a particularly effective long-term method of controlling weight.

(b) Jaw wiring

Carried out by a specialist, the patient's jaws are fixed so that normal eating and chewing is impossible. The patient must, therefore, live on a fluid diet, properly constituted to be nutritionally sound, but lower in energy than the usual diet. Jaw wiring has been used successfully on many obese people, but it has little effect on the re-education of the palate, such that the majority of patients regain weight once their jaws are released. The fixing of a nylon cord around the waist is said to help control weight gain following release of the jaws.

(c) Intestinal surgery

For many people the ideal would be to be able to eat as much as they required, but for the food not to be absorbed. Surgery to the lower gastrointestinal tract almost allows this to happen. However, the surgery brings with it many problems, not least diarrhoea and consequent electrolyte imbalance and dehydration. Patients with gross obesity which is life-threatening may be referred to specialist centres for jejuno-ileal bypass surgery.

(d) Gastroplasty and gastric banding

Many people are unable to control their appetite because they seem able to override the physiological mechanisms which tell us when we are full. In gastroplasty and gastric banding the actual size of the stomach is reduced using either staples or a band, so that only a very small quantity of food can be consumed at any one time. The volume may be reduced to 50 ml and this will obviously control the amount, but not necessarily the type of food which is eaten. Dietary advice on very small, regular meals and the use of fluid is vital to ensure a nutritionally adequate intake.

4. When should the patient be referred to the dietitian?

Many patients will manage quite well with the advice and support from the practice nurse; others will not lose any weight regardless of the amount of education and attention they are given. There will also be those who are successful for a time but whose weight then reaches a plateau and no more is lost, despite there being no change in eating habits. At this point, it is a good idea to suggest that the patient actually stops trying to diet for a short period – one or two weeks at most. This allows the patient to take their mind off the problem. Although they will eat more than they have been, many do not put on weight and those that do gain only a few pounds. After this time, the patient should attempt to diet once more. If this fails, then it may be wise to refer these patients, via their GP, to the dietitian for further advice, encouragement and support. All patients in the upper end of grade 2 and those of grade 3 obesity should be referred for specialist dietetic advice.

Remember, losing weight is not easy, but, with the proper advice and support, many people will succeed. Some of the problems which people find with dieting to lose weight and some of the suggested solutions, can be found in Chapter 9.

Chapter 3

CORONARY HEART DISEASE AND HIGH BLOOD CHOLESTEROL

Screening to identify patients with high blood cholesterol is now becoming a key feature of attempts to reduce the high prevalence of Coronary Heart Disease in the United Kingdom. While there is no "national" policy as such, many organisations, such as the British Cardiac Society and the European Atherosclerosis Society, have produced guidelines for the prevention of Coronary Heart Disease (CHD) which can be taken as the basis for local policy.

CHD is atherosclerotic arterial disease affecting the coronary arteries. The rate at which atherosclerosis develops is influenced by a number of risk factors:

- **Smoking**
- **Blood pressure**
- **Blood cholesterol**
- **Sex**
- **Weight**
- **Stress**

There are three possible strategies for prevention of CHD. The first, the population approach, involves changing risk factors in the population – information is targeted at all individuals even though some may not need it. The second involves the identification of individuals at high risk by screening systematically, for example by screening all men aged 35 to 55 years, known to have pre-existing hypertension or early death of a parent from CHD. The third is opportunistic screening: clearly within a medical practice individuals could be "caught" when an opportunity arises, for example on registering with the practice or when under review for some unrelated condition. Whatever the approach to screening there is a need for a practical management scheme to outline options available during the treatment of each individual.

Blood lipids[*]

Total blood cholesterol and LDL cholesterol are related to the risk of developing CHD – the higher the levels, the higher the risk. Having a low HDL cholesterol level can increase the risk of CHD. There is also some evidence that serum triglyceride is also a risk factor for CHD, but possibly only in some groups of people. It is thus clear that the objective of dietary management of blood lipids is to achieve optimal lipid levels; these are:

- **Total serum cholesterol**   **5.2-5.7 mmol/l**
- **LDL cholesterol**   **3.5-4.0 mmol/l**
- **Total triglyceride**   **<2.3 mmol/l**
- **HDL cholesterol**   **no defined target, probably 1.4 mmol/l**

However it must be accepted that in practice these targets may not be achieved easily. The scale of the task is illustrated in Fig. 1 taken from data reported in "The dietary and nutritional survey of British adults" (1990) which shows the distribution of total serum cholesterol for men and women aged 35–64 years: nearly 80% have values over 5.2 mmol/l, and roughly 10% are over 7.8 mmol/l.

---

[*] *see note on blood lipid metabolism at the end of this chapter.*

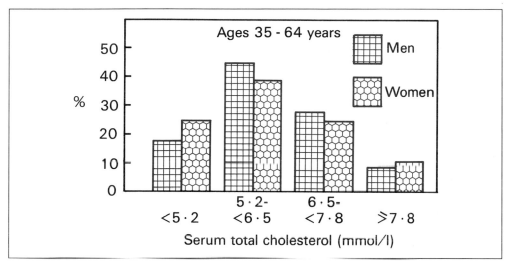

Fig. 1. The distribution of total serum cholesterol for men and women aged 35-64 years. Drawn from data reported in "The dietary and nutritional survey of British adults" (1990).

Types of hyperlipidaemia

Blood lipids may be raised due to inherent abnormalities of lipid metabolism (primary hyperlipidaemias) or secondary to other disease (secondary hyperlipidaemia).

Common causes of secondary hyperlipidaemias are:

■ **Diabetes Mellitus**

■ **Excessive alcohol intake**

■ **Hypothyroidism**

■ **Some renal diseases**

and since body weight is related to both blood cholesterol and triglyceride levels in some people:

■ **Obesity**

Primary hyperlipidaemias have been classified in various ways. The Fredrickson/WHO classification is based on pathological characteristics of the blood, but since understanding of the underlying abnormalities in primary hyperlipidaemias has developed it is now possible to classify cases according to specific defects. From this new classification, which is still evolving, come the following conditions:

49

■ **Common hypercholesterolaemia:**
the type most frequently seen, polygenic, due to raised
LDL cholesterol, not causing physical signs.

■ **Familial hypercholesterolaemia (FH):**
autosomal dominant, numbers of heterozygote cases
about 1/500 of the population, raised LDL, physical signs
(xanthomata, etc.).

■ **Familial combined hyperlipidaemia:**
raised LDL and VLDL, thus raised cholesterol and
triglyceride.

■ **Familial hypertriglyceridaemia:**
raised VLDL and chylomicrons, with physical signs (not
illustrated here).

■ **Other rarer conditions**

Most cases of raised cholesterol seen in family practice are
common hypercholesterolaemia. The other conditions are rare,
but because the blood cholesterol levels may be very high the
risk of CHD may be very great – whereas only one in 500 of the
population has the condition, amongst those who have had a
heart attack, about one in 20 has FH. Patients with FH are
likely to develop CHD and peripheral vascular disease early in
life, and it is estimated that 85% of cases are as yet undetected.
FH patients also have physical signs: xanthomata, xanthelasmata and corneal arcus, as well as signs (and symptoms) of
CHD and peripheral vascular disease early in life (see Figs.
2–4).

If physical signs are seen in patients being screened it is
appropriate to ask the family practitioner for guidance on
management. Identification of other affected family members
is also important.

Management

The following discussion is based on the management flow
chart (Fig. 5) which represents a suggested sequence of events.
Detailed thresholds for action must be discussed with the
family practitioner involved as well as the district or community dietitian.

Initial assessment

It must always be remembered that measurement of blood cholesterol is just one aspect of CHD risk factor screening – measurement of blood pressure, body weight, random or fasting blood glucose, and assessment of smoking history are all important.

A number of features may indicate that referral to the doctor for further assessment is indicated:

- **Physical signs of hyperlipidaemia:**
  these will not be common, but when present indicate the need for a full medical assessment.

- **Evidence suggestive of secondary hyperlipidaemia:**
  detection of raised fasting blood glucose, suspicion of alcohol abuse, evidence of hypothyroidism, or the existence of renal disease indicate the need for medical assessment.

- **Total blood cholesterol 7.8 mmol/l or above :**
  the family practitioner may wish to undertake a full medical review before referring back for dietary advice.

Blood cholesterol 5.2-7.8 mmol/l

If the blood cholesterol is found to be in this middle range a dietary assessment should be undertaken to determine the patient's present intake and then lipid lowering advice should be given.

The dietary assessment

The dietary assessment is best done using a printed format such as that provided in association with this book. The leaflet is reproduced in Appendix C. The patient should record all that he or she eats and drinks over a five-day period. Some patients find this easy to do, others find it difficult. Some forget to include particular items. Use of household measures does of course give only a crude assessment of intake, but it is, in fact, an effective method. In making records patients commonly:

- **Forget to record all drinks.**
- **Forget to say whether sugar was used in tea.**
- **Forget to record snacks.**

■ **Forget biscuits - the type and number eaten.**

■ **Vary in their ability to provide an accurate record - the solution is to "know your patient".**

Therefore, it is necessary to check that the diet record is as complete as possible.

Lipid lowering dietary advice

Dietary advice for lowering lipids is based on the healthy eating principles outlined in Chapter 1, however certain aspects of diet, particularly fat and soluble dietary fibre content, need to be given greater consideration.

The objectives in giving lipid lowering advice are to reduce the percentage of energy in the diet derived from fat to as near 30% as is possible (and to take only 10% from saturated fat), and to increase high carbohydrate, high fibre foods. The approach varies according to whether or not the patient is overweight or obese. If obese, then simply reducing consumption of high-fat foods will reduce energy intake and weight loss should occur. In the slim patient it is sometimes difficult to maintain weight if the patient is very concientious about cutting out fat, and perhaps because of a "small" appetite is not able to make up the energy deficit with carbohydrate foods.

Reducing fat intake is achieved by reducing consumption of:

■ **Spreading fats (butter, margarine) - by spreading thinly.**

■ **Oils - by frying rarely.**

■ **Fatty meats and meat products.**

■ **Whole milk.**

■ **Dairy products (except low fat varieties).**

■ **Nuts.**

■ **Cakes and biscuits.**

■ **Confectionery.**

The type of fat is also important .

Saturated fats, which raise blood cholesterol, should be reduced in the diet:

■ **Animal fats in**

             meat
             suet
             lard
             dairy products -   **butter**
                                    milk
                                    cheese

Polyunsaturated fats lower blood cholesterol. sometimes it may be felt appropriate to deliberately increase intake of these, especially in thin patients who would lose weight unless they were to replace some of the saturated fat with PUFA:

■ **Oils from**   **herring**
                           tuna
                           mackerel

■ **Seed oils**   **sunflower oil**
  (vegetable oils)   **corn oil**
  and margarine made **soya oil**
  from these oils

Monounsaturated fats may well be beneficial. The best source is :

Olive oil
– though rapeseed oil and groundnut oil may also be used.

It should, of course, be remembered that there is evidence that eating fatty fish (herring, tuna and mackerel) helps reduce the risk of a second heart attack in men who have already suffered from one. Fish oils are known to modify the blood clotting process – thus polyunsaturated fats are important in this respect as well as with regard to blood cholesterol.

Other dietary variables can also affect blood lipids

Dietary fibre, now broadly classified into soluble and insoluble fibre, is important. Soluble dietary fibre has been shown to lower blood cholesterol and LDL cholesterol in a number of studies, and is known to have beneficial effects on digestion and metabolism.

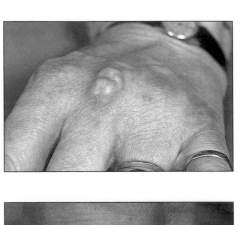

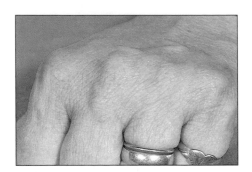

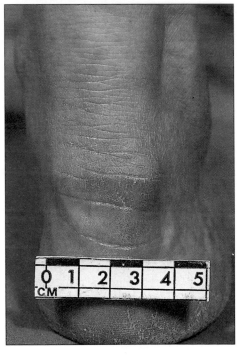

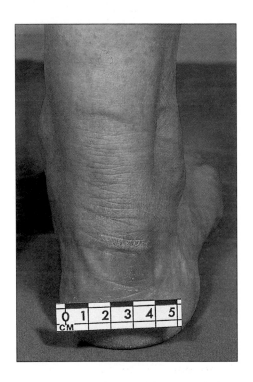

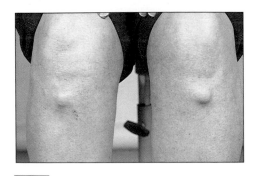

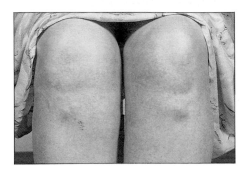

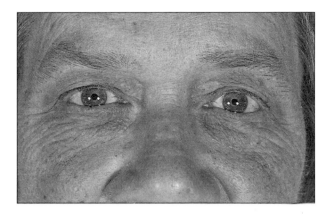

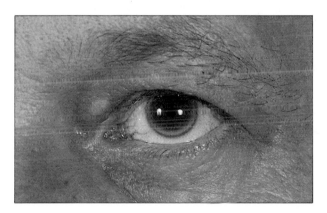

Fig. 2. (facing page). A patient with Familial Hypercholesterolaemia (FH), showing three physical signs before and after four and a half years of dietary and drug treatment. The initial total blood cholesterol was 11 5 mmol/l, which fell by 1 mmol/l with three months of lipid lowering dietary treatment; subsequent use of a lipid lowering drug (bezafibrate) reduced the level to 8.0 mmol/l. The illustrations show an extensor tendon xanthoma of the hand, an Achilles tendon xanthoma and sub-periosteal xanthomata over the tibeal tuberosity, in each case before (on the left) and after (on the right).

Fig. 3. A patient with xanthelasmata (total blood cholesterol 10.5 mmol/l)

Fig. 4. A patient with a xanthelasma and corneal arcus (total blood cholesterol 9.0 mmol/l)

Management Flow Chart for Blood Cholesterol Testing and Use of Lipid Lowering Diets in Family Practice

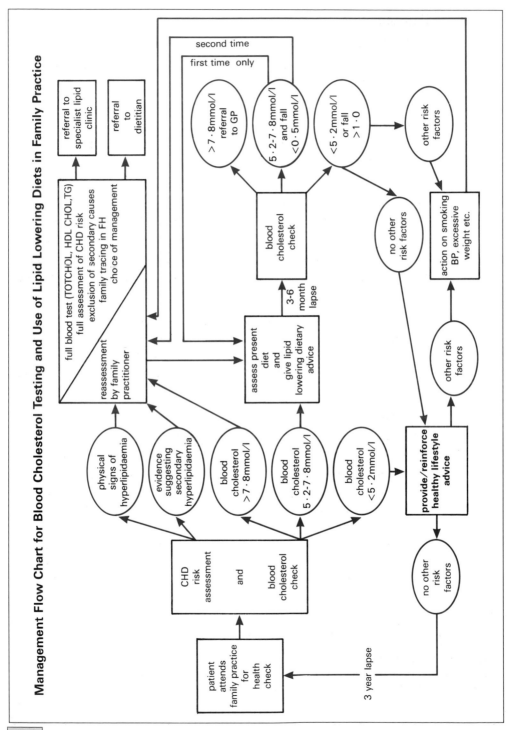

Soluble dietary fibre is found in:

- **Oats, oatmeal and oat products.**
- **Pulses (legume seeds) - peas and beans (especially chick peas and red kidney beans).**
- **Fruit.**

There is, thus, much to be gained from incorporating these foods into the lipid lowering diet. Indeed high fat foods need to be replaced with high carbohydrate, high fibre foods – oats and pulses should make a considerable contribution here.

Sugar as such may not be particularly important in the diet of patients with high blood cholesterol, unless they are over-weight in which case reduction of sugar-containing foods will help achieve weight loss. Occasionally patients with high blood triglycerides may be sensitive to dietary sugars, in which case a specific effort has to be made to minimise sugar intake.

Alcohol can also cause hypertriglyceridaemia – in such cases the need for a reduction in alcohol intake is clear, but is often difficult to achieve. In other patients alcohol contributes to dietary energy and may need to be limited especially in over-weight patients.

Patients commonly experience a number of difficulties when following a lipid lowering diet; these are:

- **they do not ask about the type of soft margarine they should be using, ie one high in polyunsaturates.**
- **they always fry in oil, thinking that oil is better than lard, but forgetting that total fat intake should be reduced.**
- **they dislike all the "right" foods and only like those they are supposed to restrict - experience is required to solve this one.**

Fig. 5. (facing page). Flow chart for the testing of blood cholesterol and use of lipid lowering diets in family practice. The thresholds and time-lapses are intended to be consistent with several current and anticipated sets of guidelines but are presented as a suggestion, not as hard and fast rules. In your practice you may choose to use different thresholds, time-lapses and management sequences.

- **they do not fully appreciate the high sugar and fat content of cakes and biscuits.**

- **they forget that sausages, pies and chicken skin are high in fat.**

- **they forget that a great variety of cheese is now available, and they need not restrict themselves to cottage cheese..**

- **they incorrectly think that they cannot eat red meat - lean cuts once or twice per week should be included.**

- **if normal or underweight, they may lose weight unless also urged to eat more starchy foods, eg potatoes, bread, pasta.**

- **they sometimes find that the cost of foods they should be buying is higher than those they would normally choose.**

Follow-up

After a lapse of three to six months blood cholesterol will be checked and those whose level has fallen to below 5.2 mmol/l or by more than 1.0 mmol/l may be given healthy lifestyle advice and be reviewed in three years, unless there are other risk factors which require attention. Those whose lipids remain in the range 5.2–7.8 mmol/l or whose level has fallen less than 0.5 mmol/l should be reassessed and given reinforcement of lipid lowering dietary advice. If, on further checking of the blood cholesterol there has been no improvement, consultation with the family practitioner is suggested – at this time, referral to the dietitian may be appropriate.

Blood cholesterol under 5.2 mmol/l

Those found on screening to have blood cholesterol levels under 5.2 mmol/l should be given healthy lifestyle advice, as well as advice related to any other risk factors. If all is well, a follow-up health screening would ideally occur three years later.

Target levels for blood lipids

While target levels for blood lipids may be correct on the basis of association with risk, a total blood cholesterol fall as a result of dietary change in a normal weight individual is unlikely to

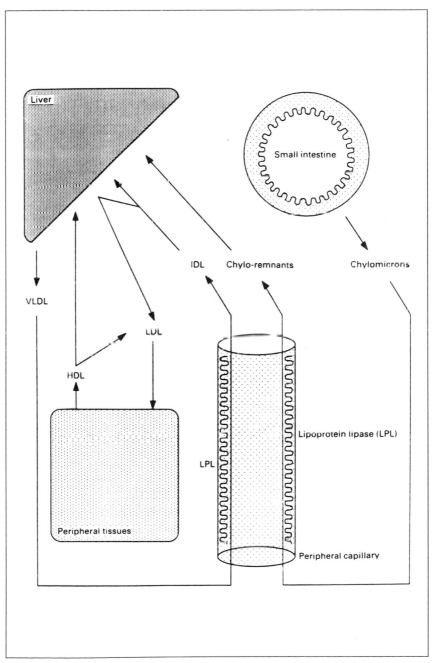

Fig. 6. Figure illustrating some aspects of cholesterol metabolism (see text). Reproduced with permission from "Complex carbohydrates in foods – report of a British Nutrition Foundation Task Force" published by Chapman & Hall, London, 1990.

exceed 1.0 mmol/l. Thus the level in a patient with a starting value of 7.8 mmol/l may, even after a good starting response, be as high as 6.8 mmol/l. If such an individual has no other risk factors there is probably little merit in attempting further lipid reduction – few doctors would use drugs in such a case. If, however, such an individual had a very strong family history of CHD, or was known to have a very low HDL cholesterol, then careful consideration would have to be given to the case.

A note on blood lipid metabolism (see Fig. 6)

Dietary cholesterol and dietary fat (as triglyceride) are incorporated into chylomicrons in the small intestinal wall. Chylomicrons then pass in the blood stream to peripheral capillaries where they are broken down by lipoprotein-lipase; the fat (triglyceride) is taken up by cells in the peripheral tissue, leaving chylomicron remnants containing cholesterol which are taken up by the liver. Cholesterol is also secreted by the liver in very low density lipoprotein (VLDL) particles, which also contain a lot of triglyceride fat. These particles are also broken down in the peripheral capillaries, again releasing triglyceride into the peripheral tissues, leaving in this case intermediate density (IDL) particles. Some IDL is taken up by the liver, some is converted to low-density lipoprotein (LDL), which in turn is taken up mainly by the liver, but also by peripheral tissues. High density lipoprotein (HDL) synthesised in the liver or small intestine transports cholesterol from peripheral tissue to the liver or by transfer to other particles.

Chapter 4

HYPERTENSION

Blood pressure control

Blood pressure fluctuates between two extremes which correspond to the filling of the left ventricle of the heart (diastolic – low pressure) and the ejection of the blood into the arteries (systolic – high pressure). Blood pressure (BP) is controlled by nervous and hormonal mechanisms which interact at many points. The key organ linking these functions is the kidney, which controls water and sodium excretion.

It is important to maintain blood pressure in order to supply blood to the tissues, especially the brain. However, if the BP rises too high, blood vessels may be damaged.

Hypertension

It is difficult to define normal and high blood pressure for individuals in the UK as, in common with many other Western populations, blood pressure increases with age. The average blood pressure in a group of people varies from 120/80 mmHg (systolic/diastolic) at the age of 20 to 160/90 mmHg at 60, an approximate increase of 10 mmHg for every 10 years of age. Hypertension must, therefore, be defined as a blood pressure above the average value for the patient's age group. The World Health Organization defines hypertension as a systolic BP above 160 mmHg and/or a diastolic BP above 95 mmHg. Many practices will have specific protocols for treating patients – if

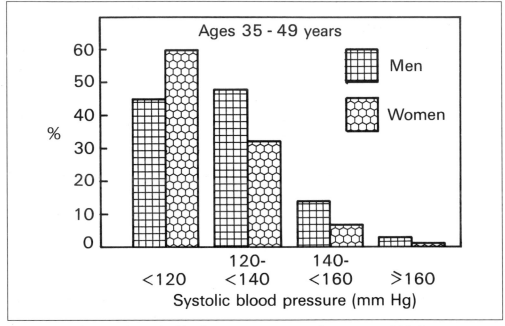

Fig. 1. Distribution of systolic blood pressure in men and women aged 35-49 years. Data derived from "The dietary and nutritional survey of British adults", J Gregory et al, OPCS, HMSO, 1990. The survey work was undertaken in 1986 and 1987.
Fig. 2. Distribution of diastolic blood pressure in men and women aged 35-49 years. Data derived from "The dietary and nutritional survey of British adults" (see above).

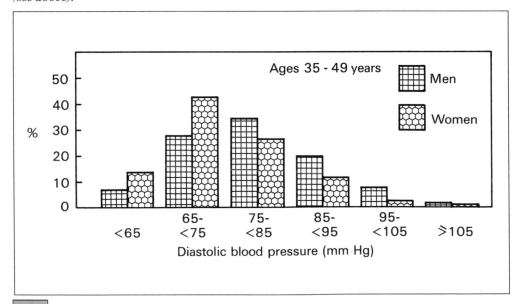

you do not, the flow chart (Fig. 3) may serve as a basis for discussion. Depending on the age of your patient and other risk factors, you may decide that some of the general health education measures, such as weight loss, limitation of alcohol intake and stress management, need to be instituted even though BP is only marginally raised. For example, in a 40 year old man who is overweight and has a family history of hypertension, you might want to suggest changes even though his diastolic BP is only 90.

The scale of the problem in the community is illustrated in Figs. 1 & 2, which indicate that perhaps 1 in 10 men and 1 in 20 women between the ages of 35 and 49 may need treatment for hypertension.

Primary and secondary hypertension

It is possible to divide hypertension into two basic types: PRIMARY (or ESSENTIAL) and SECONDARY. Primary hypertension is by far the most common and is estimated to represent between 80–95% of cases of hypertension. Secondary hypertension is the consequence of other medical conditions, such as kidney disease or some forms of heart disease. The patient with secondary hypertension must obviously receive treatment for the causal conditions, management of which will not be discussed here.

Primary hypertension probably has no single cause but is multifactorial in origin. Factors which may be involved are:

- **Heredity - family history is important.**
- **Gender - women may be protected by hormonal factors before the menopause, but are more susceptible afterwards.**
- **Diet - especially excessive salt intake.**
- **Obesity.**
- **Stress.**

Almost all hypotheses about high BP suggest that inability of the kidney to cope with excess intakes of sodium is important. Another idea is that some people with hypertension have an unbalanced nervous control of blood pressure (overactivity of the sympathetic nervous system). Prolonged exposure to high blood pressure together with factors related to ageing (athero-sclerosis or calcification of the arteries) may also contribute to high blood pressure by altering the elasticity of the arterial wall and by affecting the sensitivity of the baro-receptors.

Problems

Primary hypertension is often asymptomatic, but the patient may complain of headaches and failing vision. The benefits of treating mild or borderline hypertension are controversial, but there is some agreement that the detection and treatment of symptomless hypertension is worthwhile and many GP prac-tices will be involved in screening the middle-aged population.

Moderately severe hypertension (diastolic pressure 105 mmHg) should always be treated. The long-term effects of untreated hypertension are higher risks of heart disease and stroke, congestive cardiac failure and possibly also renal failure, retinopathy and hypertensive encephalopathy.

If, on screening, the patient's BP is apparently high, it is a good idea to repeat the measurement after he or she has rested for a while and when you are sure that he or she is at ease with you. BP is sometimes raised simply because the person is nervous. If it is consistently raised, then discussion with the doctor should decide the course of action. If the diastolic BP is above 100 mmHg, it is probable that further investigations such as urinalysis, plasma urea and electrolytes and plasma lipids may be necessary to exclude any underlying cause. If the diastolic BP is greater than 105 mmHg, this should be dis-cussed with the doctor immediately as the patient will almost certainly need rapid investigation and treatment. See manage-ment flow chart (Fig. 3).

Dietary factors in hypertension

In the patient with mild or moderate hypertension, diet will probably be an important part of the treatment and in some

Fig. 3. (facing page). Flow chart for the testing of blood pressure and use of diet in family practice. The thresholds and time-lapses presented here are suggestions rather than hard and fast rules. In your practice you may choose to use different thresholds, time-lapses and management sequences.

Management Flow Chart for Blood Pressure Testing and Use of Diet in Family Practice

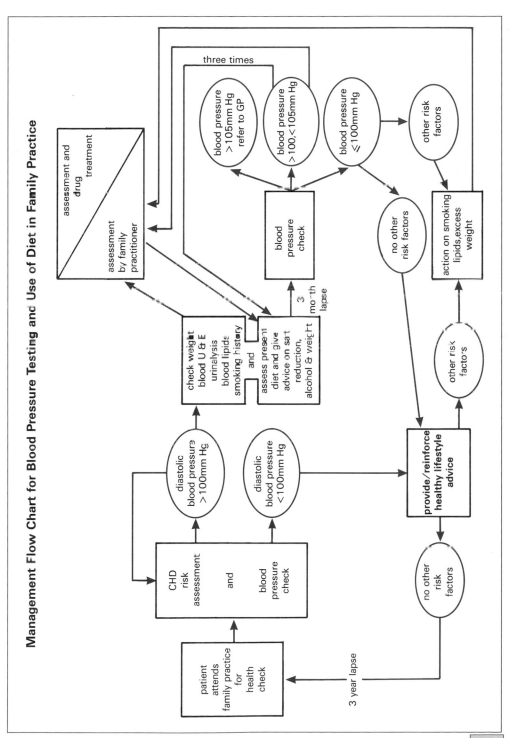

cases the only treatment. Even when antihypertensive drugs are necessary, the patient's diet may also be important – for example, it has been shown that ACE inhibitors are more effective if salt in the diet is reduced.

Several diet-related factors have been suggested to be important in hypertension. The most important are:

- **Obesity - weight reduction will often bring down high BP.**
- **Sodium intake - excess sodium increases BP in susceptible patients.**
- **Potassium intake - a low intake may increase BP.**

In addition, there is a suggestion that low calcium intake may exacerbate hypertension and recent evidence suggests that a high intake of polyunsaturated fatty acids (PUFA) and dietary fibre may reduce blood pressure. These ideas are still quite controversial. However, if you advise your patients about general "healthy eating", you will automatically be advising them to increase fibre and probably PUFA at the same time.

Treatment of mild to moderate hypertension

1. Weight control

If patients are overweight, they should be encouraged to follow a suitable reducing diet based on the healthy eating suggestions in Chapter 1.

Weight reduction alone will often result in a significant fall in BP.

2. Sodium intake

Sodium in food is mainly in the form of sodium chloride – common salt. Most people take much more salt than they need, but you should find out if the patient is in this group before advising to cut down. Many people are not aware that there is hidden salt in foods and will feel that they do not have much salt simply because they do not add it to cooked foods. However, it has been estimated that over 80% of the sodium in the UK diet comes from processed foods.

Table 1 outlines some of the sources of salt in the diet.

Table 1: Foods with high sodium content

Table salt, bicarbonate of soda and any foods containing these.

Bacon, ham, gammon, sausages, beefburgers (unless home-made), tinned meat, meat pastes and patés.

Smoked or tinned fish, eg smoked haddock, cod, mackerel, kippers, fish in brine, fish pastes & patés, shell fish.

Cheese, especially blue cheese.

Meat or yeast extracts and stock cubes.

Tinned vegetables, baked beans, spaghetti in tomato sauce. All bottled sauces, ketchup, chutney, salad cream.

Salted savoury or cheese biscuits.

Crisps, salted or roast peanuts, other savoury snacks.

Proprietary indigestion preparations containing sodium bicarbonate should be avoided, eg liver salts or bicarbonate of soda itself. Aluminium or magnesium hydroxide based products could be recommended instead.

Table 2: Salt substitutes

Salt substitutes containing potassium or ammonium salts are usually allowed, eg Selora, Ruthmol.

Other products are lower in sodium but still contain considerable amounts, eg Lo-salt.

Sea salt contains traces of other minerals but has almost as much sodium as ordinary salt.

The following simple questions should give you some idea about whether the patient has a high intake of salt:

- **Do you add salt at table before tasting your food?**
- **Do you use salt in cooking?**
- **Do you eat salty foods such as cheese, bacon, ham, smoked or salted fish more than three times a week?**
- **Do you eat canned meats or vegetables more than once or twice each week?**
- **Do you use bottled sauces and pickles regularly?**

If the person answers yes to three or more of these questions, it is probable that their salt intake is quite high. The majority of people in this country eat far more salt than they really need and can easily cut down with some simple advice.

If you find that your patient is at his ideal weight or has managed to reduce to a sensible weight and does not have a high salt intake but still has a diastolic pressure over 100 mmHg, then he should be referred back to the doctor.

Advice for reducing sodium

The person should be advised to use only a small amount of salt in cooking, eg a pinch in a pan of vegetables for four people, and should not add salt at table.

Intake of the highly salted foods listed in Table 1 should be limited to two or three portions a week: the patient leaflet explains this in more detail.

People who are used to highly salted foods often find reducing salt intake difficult at first, but should be encouraged to persist. It has been shown that perseverance will often result in a reduced taste for salt. Herbs and spices are useful for flavouring foods and a useful low salt cookery book is listed in Appendix 5.

Potassium intake

Potassium is found in all foods, but is especially abundant in fruits and vegetables. Where financial circumstances allow, there is no harm in advising that the patient eats at least two portions of these every day. Potatoes are a good source of potassium as well and unless patients are limiting intake to help control weight, they should be encouraged to eat them. Potatoes are a cheaper source of potassium if the patient cannot afford to buy lots of fruit.

Some patients may ask about salt substitutes if they don't like the taste of unsalted food and these are usually high in potassium. See Table 2.

BEWARE – patients with hypertension due to kidney disease may not be allowed a high potassium diet and the advice above is then not appropriate – they should discuss this with their dietitian.

Alcohol

The "safe" limit for alcohol intake for healthy men and women is said to be 21 and 14 units per week respectively, but this is excessive for the person with hypertension. High alcohol intake may increase the risk of raised BP and the hypertensive patient should use alcohol as an occasional treat.

A standard drink is equivalent to:

- 1/2 pint of beer, cider or lager.
- 1 measure of spirits.
- 1 small glass of wine or sherry

Alcohol is contra-indicated with many anti-hypertensive drugs.

Non-dietary factors

1. Stress may exacerbate hypertension and while a certain amount of stress cannot be avoided patients may need advice on how to slow down the pace of life and learn to relax. Relaxation techniques have been used successfully by doctors to treat hypertensive patients and avoid drug treatment. Some people find that exercise, such as walking or swimming, helps them.

The very anxious patient may need sedation.

2. All patients should be encouraged not to smoke and if they do smoke should be helped to plan a programme to help them stop.

Treatment of severe hypertension

In severe hypertension, attention to the dietary and lifestyle factors above, together with antihypertensive drugs will usually achieve acceptable control of BP. The drugs will usually have to be taken indefinitely.

Chapter 5

DIABETES MELLITUS

1. What is it?

The hormone insulin is secreted by the β-cells of the Islets of Langerhans in the pancreas and is essential for the normal uptake of glucose by the tissues. Diabetes mellitus is the result of either a complete lack of insulin or an ineffective use of insulin.

If insulin is not secreted or its use is ineffective, then levels of glucose in the blood will rise. Once this rise exceeds the renal threshold, glucose will spill out into the urine where it can be detected. The hyperglycaemia and glycosuria then give rise to the main symptoms of diabetes of which most patients complain before diagnosis:

- ■ Polyuria
- ■ Polydipsia
- ■ Weight loss
- ■ Lethargy

Diabetes my also present as a result of infection, or other illness, and may also be found on routine testing.

(1) Insulin dependent diabetes (IDDM)

This type of diabetes occurs mainly in young people, but can also occur in later life. Patients produce little or no insulin and so are dependent on exogenous insulin to live.

(2) Non-insulin dependent diabetes (NIDDM)

This occurs mainly in older overweight people and is the most prevalent form of the disorder. There is also an increased risk in some ethnic minority groups. These patients produce some insulin and so are not dependent on exogenous insulin to live.

Diabetes cannot be cured, but it can be well controlled in the majority of patients using diet, either alone or with oral hypoglycaemic drugs or insulin.

2. Diagnosis

The majority of patients present to their general practitioner with one or more of the symptoms outlined above. Only a minority of cases will present as a medical emergency in diabetic coma.

Initial diagnosis is often made by testing the urine for the presence of glucose and taking blood for an estimation of blood glucose (Table 1).

3. Treatment

The treatment of diabetes has three main aims:

- **To keep blood glucose levels as near to normal limits as possible, preventing both hyperglycaemia and hypoglycaemia as well as wide swings in levels.**
- **To maintain optimum nutrition and to achieve and maintain optimum weight.**
- **To delay the onset of the complications of the disorder for as long as possible.**

In order to achieve these aims, frequent urine glucose or capillary blood glucose tests should be done.

In the non-diabetic, blood glucose levels range between 3–8 mmol/l, rising shortly after meals and then decreasing. While it would be ideal for all diabetics to attain this level of blood glucose, it is not practically possible. The fasting blood glucose levels shown in Table 2 may be taken as indicating the current state of the diabetes.

Table 1. Diagnostic values for blood glucose levels in diabetes

	GLUCOSE CONCENTRATION mmol/l			
	Whole blood		Plasma	
	venous	capillary	venous	capillary
Unstandardized (casual, random)				
Diabetes likely	≥10.0	≥11.1	≥11.1	≥12.2
Diabetes unlikely	≤4.4	≤4.4	≤5.5	≤5.5
(range between figures given represents the uncertain zone)				
Fasting*	≥6.7	>6.7	≥7.8	≥7.8
2 h after 75 g oral glucose*	≥10.0	≥11.1	≥11.1	≥12.2

(* figures diagnostic for diabetes mellitus)

Table 2. Fasting blood glucose level

< 3 mmol/l	hypoglycaemia
3 - 8 mmol/l	good control
8 - 13 mmol/l	fair control
> 13 mmol/l	poor control

However, it is important to remember that measuring blood glucose levels is not an indicator of long-term diabetic control – ie it does not tell us anything about the diabetic control over the previous, say, six weeks.

A much better measure of long-term control is an estimation of the level of glycosylated haemoglobin, HbA_{1c}. The normal HbA_{1c} level is 5–8%, though values differ between laboratories.

Ideally all diabetics should have levels within this range and the following example is for values from one particular laboratory:

Table 3. HbA$_{1c}$ level	
5 - 8 %	very good control
8 - 10 %	good control
10 - 12 %	fair control
> 12 %	poor control

Patients may also be asked to test their urine regularly and record the results on a chart. The amount of glucose in the urine at any one time is not a true reflection of the amount in the blood for the urine will have been collecting for some hours. However, urine testing may be a useful tool in assessing control over time, particularly in the older non-insulin dependent diabetic.

Diet

The dietary treatment of diabetes has changed considerably since the publication by the British Diabetic Association in 1983 of a paper outlining dietary recommendations for diabetics. At around the same time, the National Advisory Committee on Nutrition Education (NACNE) published guidelines on diet for the general population. These two sets of guidelines were very similar such that the diabetic diet is now based upon the healthy eating guidelines for the general population – high in fibre and low in fat and sugar. These guidelines are set out in detail in Appendix 1.

The initial dietary education of the diabetic should have been carried out by the dietitian. The practice nurse role will be to reinforce this education, to try to solve any dietary problems and to monitor weight and diabetic control. It is important that any problems with which the nurse cannot deal adequately are referred to the dietitian. Such problems might include unexplained weight gain, consistently raised blood glucose or lipids, or problems with specific items of diet.

The aims of the dietary treatment are to:

■ **Achieve near normal blood levels of glucose and lipids.**

■ **Minimize the risk of hypoglycaemia in diabetics treated with insulin and certain hypoglycaemic drugs.**

■ **Reduce and/or maintain body weight.**

Oral hypoglycaemic drugs

There are two types of oral hypoglycaemic drugs (OHGs) used to control diabetes in Britain.

(1) The sulphonylureas

These act by stimulating the pancreas to produce more insulin. The newer, or second generation, sulphonylureas are less potent than the older drugs. This means that it is less likely now for a patient taking these drugs to become hypoglycaemic under certain circumstances (particularly if a meal is missed), than was the case in the past. Nevertheless, patients will need to be told the importance of eating regular meals which contain carbohydrates and how to recognize and treat a hypoglycaemic reaction. It is not uncommon for patients taking sulphonylureas to gain weight.

(2) The biguanides

The action of the biguanides is to make the insulin which the patient produces more effective. There is only one biguanide – Metformin – now available in Britain. Metformin is useful on its own for the overweight diabetic, but may also be prescribed with a sulphonylurea where a non-insulin dependent diabetic is poorly controlled.

Biguanides do not produce hypoglycaemia, but they may cause gastrointestinal disturbance.

Insulin

Insulin is a protein and so would be broken down by digestion were it taken in by mouth. Therefore exogenous insulin must be injected subcutaneously. The different kinds of insulin have varying modes of action and the number of injections per day depends upon the type of insulin taken.

It is important that the insulin regimen for any one patient is chosen to fit in with the patient's diet and lifestyle. Increasingly, insulin dependent diabetics are being treated with short acting insulin, given via a pen system, three or more times each day before meals. An injection of long acting insulin is also necessary to cover background physiological needs.

Pregnancy in diabetic women needs special care – consult with your local dietitians. Such consultation should, of course, take place concerning gestational diabetes, which is fairly common, especially in Asian minority groups.

In some cases, often pregnant diabetics, or poorly controlled young diabetics, patients may take their insulin via a pump system. This involves the implantation of a small needle attached to a length of tubing subcutaneously, usually in the abdomen. The tubing is then attached to a pump containing insulin in a syringe. The pump can be set to provide a constant small dose of insulin to cover physiological needs and to introduce a larger dose of insulin just before meals. Both the pen injector and the pump give better control of diabetes because they mimic the normal physiological state.

Diet-specific variables

(**a**) **Energy:** Achieving the correct dietary energy (Calorie) intake for each individual remains the most important feature of dietary management. Maintaining a steady body weight, or achieving weight loss (discussed below and in Chapter 2) is clearly dependent on getting the right Calorie intake.

(**b**) **Sources of energy:** Fat, carbohydrate, and protein provide the energy (Calories) in the diet. The protein content of the diet is not usually deliberately changed, though recently evidence has been produced showing that the development of kidney problems in diabetics may be slowed by limiting dietary protein. If any of your patients are prescribed such a diet please discuss details with your local dietitians.

■ **Fat:**

The diabetic diet should be low in total fat because of the increased risk of cardiovascular disease. For the same reason, the diet should be high in polyunsaturated fats. The chapter on hyperlipidaemia explains the different effects of various dietary fats on blood lipids. In practice, the diabetic should be encouraged not to spread too much fat on bread and not to fry foods too often. Spreading fat should be polyunsaturated margarine or low fat spread, and cooking oils should also contain PUFA. These fats should also be used for baking. Semi-skimmed milk is suitable if the diabetic finds skimmed milk unacceptable. Hard cheeses should be kept to a minimum.

■ **Carbohydrate – fibre and sugar:**

There are two types of dietary fibre, soluble and insoluble. These are found in different foods and each type of fibre has a different function. Soluble fibre is found in oats, oat bran, oat products, and vegetables, especially pulse vegetables and fruit. It is especially important to the diabetic because it slows the post-prandial rise in blood glucose levels. It also has a beneficial effect on blood lipid levels, lowering total and LDL blood cholesterol. Insoluble fibre is found in cereal foods other than oats. Although its effect on blood glucose levels is not as marked as soluble fibre, foods containing insoluble fibre are still important in the diabetic diet. Diabetics should, therefore, be encouraged to eat:

- ■ **Wholemeal or other high fibre breads.**
- ■ **Oats, oat products and oat cereals.**
- ■ **Wholemeal pasta and cereals, and brown rice.**
- ■ **Pulses, eg lentils, red kidney beans, peas, baked beans.**
- ■ **Fruit – with skin where appropriate.**
- ■ **Vegetables – with skin where appropriate, including potatoes.**

Porridge is an ideal breakfast dish. Main meals should be accompanied by plenty of vegetables, with a pudding consisting of fruit – either fresh or tinned in natural juice. The old system of "counting" exchanges of fruit and vegetables, bread and cereals is regarded as less important now.

Diabetics must be advised to increase their fluid intake as they increase their fibre intake. At least eight cups of fluid per day should be taken.

The British Diabetic Association suggests that sugar intake should be limited to 25 g per day, which should be taken as part of fibre-containing meals. Recent research has shown that sugar and sugar-containing foods have less of an effect on blood glucose if they are eaten as part of a fibre-containing meal. Nevertheless, excessive use of sugar is contraindicated and the BDA recommendation should still be followed. Artificial sweeteners are useful in drinks (see Chapter 2).

(c) Alcohol: All diabetics should be aware of the fact that alcohol has a hypoglycaemic effect. It is, therefore, important that the diabetic does not drink alcohol on an empty stomach. They should also be aware of the differing alcohol contents of the variety of beers now available, in particular those marketed as low in carbohydrate. These beers are actually **higher** in alcohol than ordinary beers and should be avoided. Beers which are marketed as low in alcohol or alcohol-free still contain sugar and hence energy. Under no circumstances should a diabetic drink and drive.

(d) Salt: Excessive salt consumption should be discouraged, especially if the diabetic is also hypertensive. A diet which is high in fibre and low in fat will be naturally lower in salt than a diet consisting of a lot of convenience food. However, it would be wise to check on the consumption of foods, such as bacon, ham and smoked meats and fish, and on the amount of salt which is added both in cooking and at table. It will do no harm to suggest that the diabetic stops adding salt to food at table.

Diet - general considerations

(a) Insulin dependent diabetes: Traditionally, insulin dependent diabetics have been managed in hospital diabetic clinics by consultants, physicians, and dietitians. After the initial education by the dietitian, follow-up management is increasingly carried out in general practice in close association with the specialist diabetes nurse and the dietitian.

Meals should be spread evenly throughout the day and between meal snacks should be encouraged to minimize hypoglycaemia. Timing of all meals and snacks must fit in with individual lifestyles. Complex fibre-containing carbohydrate foods should be taken at all meals and snacks, and there is no need to avoid sugar-containing foods completely, though sugar intake should still be restricted.

It is important to stress that the insulin dependent diabetic does not miss meals or snacks. This is important regardless of the insulin regimen. Those diabetics who take their insulin by injection twice each day will need to be eating at regular times in order that a relatively constant supply of glucose is delivered to the blood. Any change in weight, diabetic control or blood lipid levels should indicate a referral to the dietitian.

(b) Non-insulin dependent diabetes: The dietary treatment will depend upon the patient's weight.

■ **The normal weight non-insulin dependent diabetic** will require a diet similar to that of the insulin dependent diabetic, based upon their energy requirements. If their current diet keeps their weight stable, then converting that diet using basic healthy eating principles will be all that is required.

The patient might be asked to complete a food diary from time to time in order that the nurse can keep a check on the diet. Any sudden change in weight, blood sugar, blood lipid levels, or diabetic control should indicate that more specialist advice might be required and the patient should be referred to the dietitian.

■ **The overweight non-insulin dependent diabetic.** Those patients who are overweight should be encouraged to try to reduce their weight to normal. The advice for reducing weight as given in Chapter 2 will be equally suitable for the overweight non-insulin dependent diabetic. Patients can be encouraged to keep to the diet by reinforcement of the message that their diabetic symptoms may disappear once their excess weight is lost. However, it is important that the patients do not get the message that their diabetes will "go away" if they lose weight. They must understand that they will need to adopt new eating habits for life, not just until their urine is free from sugar and their blood glucose levels are normal. The patients should be treated in the same way as the obese in the first instance.

(c) Special diabetic foods: Diabetic chocolate, biscuits and jams are expensive and unnecessary, though it is often difficult to convince patients of this fact! With the slight relaxation of the view on sugar intake described above, diabetics may occasionally eat ordinary preserves on their bread, ordinary biscuits, even chocolate-covered ones especially if they contain fibre, and may eat sweets and chocolate as part of or after their meals. Low calorie or "diet" fizzy drinks and squashes are extremely useful and there is a wide variety now available. Fruits tinned in natural juice are superior to those tinned in sorbitol or fructose syrup, more widely available, and cheaper.

Exercise

The diabetic should be encouraged to exercise as a means of keeping weight stable and helping diabetic control.

An increase in carbohydrate intake before exercise is necessary because the exercise increases the uptake of glucose by the muscles, resulting in a lower blood glucose.

The amount of extra carbohydrate will be different depending upon the individual and the type of exercise. Short bursts of fairly strenuous activity will require a sugary food or drink to be taken before the exercise. More prolonged exercise, which may be more gentle, is better supported by a starchy carbohydrate which will be released more slowly.

Snack suggestions

Strenuous exercise:

Mini chocolate bar, eg Mars, Milky Way; or a couple of chocolate biscuits.

Prolonged exercise:

2–3 digestive biscuits; piece of fruit and plain biscuit; fruit, yoghurt and plain biscuit; piece of fruit and packet of nuts and raisins.

A snack of easily assimilable carbohydrate, eg chocolate or glucose tablets, should be available to the diabetic during and after exercise. It may also be necessary to have some carbohydrate at the next meal.

Hypoglycaemia

All diabetic patients on Sulphonylureas or Insulin treatment are at risk of hypoglycaemia (blood glucose <2.5 mmol/l). They should thus be given appropriate instructions on how to cope with the condition.

Causes of hypoglycaemia:

insulin treated patients	*sulphonylurea treated patients*
too much insulin	tablet overdose
not enough food	not enough food
a delayed meal	unusual exercise
unusual exercise	vomiting
stress	

Frequent episodes of hypoglycaemia usually indicate that a change of treatment is indicated.

Signs of hypoglycaemia

excessive sweating	faintness
paleness	headache
tingling of lips	pounding of the heart
blurred vision	hunger
irritability	lack of concentration
personality change	not able to be awakened

Sugar or food containing sugar should be given immediately (eg two heaped teaspoonsful of sugar in a drink, or three glucose tablets) followed by biscuits, or yoghurt or a sandwich. Glucagon may be issued to close relatives of insulin treated patients, for use in an emergency. However thorough teaching on use of glucagon must be given before it is issued.

Management of illness

Any illness and especially infective disease will affect diabetic control. Where the illness is short lived the disturbance of control will matter very little provided that the patient is not insulin treated. In such non-insulin treated patients, once the illness has passed and the patient is able to return to normal life and food intake, control will return. In the insulin dependent diabetic and the diabetic taking oral hypoglycaemic drugs, an illness which affects the appetite can be difficult to manage.

Insulin dependent diabetics

Uncontrolled vomiting in a patient with insulin dependent diabetes is a serious condition which requires immediate medical attention.

Insulin dependent diabetics must never stop using insulin.

In all cases of infection, vomiting or any other illness the blood glucose should be tested frequently and the insulin dosage increased if necessary. Medical assistance should be obtained if the illness continues for more than 24 hours.

Test the urine for ketones.

If the patient cannot eat then carbohydrate in the usual diet can be replaced with fluid or semi-solid alternatives.

Diabetics treated with oral hypoglycaemic drugs

If the patient is vomiting, the tablets should not be taken, the urine sugar and/or blood glucose should be tested frequently and sugar-free drinks should be given. If the blood glucose or urine sugar remain high, or the vomiting continues for more than 24 hours medical attention should be obtained. In other illnesses sulphonylureas should be continued. If necessary replace solid food with easily absorbed carbohydrate, but if there are any uncertainties seek medical advice.

Suitable foods to be used during illness

Normal meals should be replaced by taking approximately 10 g carbohydrate as a semi-solid or fluid food every hour (some suggestions are given below). As the patient begins to feel better then this may be increased to 20g carbohydrate two hourly until appetite returns and light foods are tolerated.

The following foods contain about 10g carbohydrate:

> **2 teaspoonsful sugar or glucose (dissolved in water)**
>
> **2 desertspoons of Complan in water**
>
> **1 teaspoonful honey or sugar dissolved in low calorie squash**
>
> **1 tablespoonful Ribena diluted in water**
>
> **1/3 pint milk**
>
> **4 oz pure fruit juice (diluted if necessary)**
>
> **1 plain yoghurt or half a flavoured yoghurt**
>
> **1/3 pint cream soup (eg tomato or chicken soup)**

Summary

The diabetic diet is identical to the healthy diet outlined in Chapter 1. Special foods are not necessary and the diabetic does not need to eat food which is any different from that eaten by the rest of the family. Overweight diabetics should be encouraged to reduce their weight to normal, which is important for their long-term control. The practice nurse has a vital role to play in the continuing education and support of the diabetic patient.

Chapter 6

DIET AND THE RISK OF CANCER

Although great advances have been made in the early diagnosis and treatment of cancer, about one in four deaths in the United Kingdom are due to cancer. Environmental factors have long been known to play a part in the causation of some cancers: diet is believed to be a causative factor in as many as one in three cases of cancer. The evidence linking dietary factors and some types of cancer is derived from comparisons of diet and cancer rates between countries, and between groups within countries, especially immigrant groups whose dietary habits may change over a generation or two. Study of the diets of those who have developed cancer, compared to those who have not, has also given clues. Huge studies of large numbers of people over several decades are now underway to provide more evidence in the future, when it may be possible to give more detailed guidelines. For the time being the evidence available allows the advice described below to be given, but it must not be forgotten that the evidence linking smoking to cancer and exposure to sunlight to skin cancer is much stronger than the evidence relating dietary factors to cancer.

Specific dietary factors

Alcohol

Alcohol consumption is clearly linked to cancer of the oral cavity, pharynx, larynx, oesophagus and liver. In Britain these cancers are not as common as in other countries where alcohol consumption levels are higher. Nevertheless even moderate drinking is linked to higher risk and the combination of heavy smoking and heavy drinking leads to a very greatly increased risk of oral cancer

Fat

There is some evidence for a link between dietary fat and breast and large bowel cancer, but also some evidence which does not support this link. Reducing fat in the diet is clearly indicated in some people in order to reduce risk of coronary heart disease. In such individuals it is possible that the dietary change may also be of benefit in reducing cancer risk.

Obesity

Obesity is associated with increased risks of some cancers and decreased risks of others. The risk of breast cancer in postmenopausal women is increased if the individual is obese.

Fruit and vegetables

People who eat a relatively large amount of fruit and vegetables seem to be at lower risk of developing cancer of the stomach, oesophagus, large bowel and lung, compared with those who eat little. Nutrients contained in vegetables – eg vitamin C, beta- carotene and other carotenoids, vitamin E, and riboflavin – have been shown to reduce cancer risk under some experimental circumstances, but other, as yet unidentified, constituents of fruit and vegetables may be important.

Dietary fibre

There is no clear evidence that dietary fibre protects against large bowel cancer, but there is an enormous scientific literature which suggests that it might do. It must be remembered that when fat in the diet is reduced in quantity it is replaced with high carbohydrate, high fibre foods, unless the patient is trying to lose weight. Such a change may in the future be proved to reduce the risk of large bowel cancer.

Meat, protein and salt

The evidence linking these variables with cancer risk is not sufficient to allow clear recommendations to be made. It must, however, be remembered that salt consumption is usually far in excess of that needed to meet physiological requirement. Reduction of intake rarely does any harm and may be shown, in future, to be beneficial.

Smoked, cured, pickled and barbecued foods

Evidence linking consumption of these foods with cancer, and the high content of substances believed to be cancer-causing in some foods processed in these ways, suggests that it would be unwise to increase consumption of these foods.

Specific nutrients

Vitamin A and beta-carotene

Early work suggested that those who ate higher amounts of foods containing vitamin A were protected to some extent from some cancers, especially lung cancer. The view now, however, is that it is more likely to be the precursor substance, beta-carotene, from which vitamin A is synthesised in the gut, which is the protective agent. Beta-carotene is one of a group of substances, the carotenoids, some of which may be more protective against cancer than beta-carotene. Beta-carotene, unlike vitamin A, has not been demonstrated to be toxic at high doses, but a range of carotenoids are best acquired by eating more fruit and vegetables.

Vitamins C and E and selenium

Evidence exists linking intake levels of these three nutrients and risk of cancer. There are sound reasons for expecting them to play a role in modifying cancer risk, but as yet insufficient evidence on which to base a specific recommendation. Excessive intake of selenium, and to a lesser extent vitamin C, is dangerous, and the best safe option at present is, again, to increase consumption of fruit and vegetables.

European Code Against Cancer

Using all the evidence linking dietary and other factors with cancer, a set of recommendations has been prepared by the committee of cancer experts of the European Community. The Code is as follows:

Certain cancers may be avoided if you:

- **1. Do not smoke.**
- **2. Moderate your consumption of alcoholic drinks.**
- **3. Avoid excessive exposure to the sun.**
- **4. Follow health and safety instructions, especially concerning production, handling or use of any substance which may cause cancer.**

Your general health will benefit if you do the following:

- **5. Frequently eat fresh fruits, vegetables and high fibre cereals.**
- **6. Avoid becoming overweight and limit your intake of fatty foods.**

More cancers will be cured if detected early, hence:

- **7. See a doctor if you notice a lump, or observe a change in a mole, or abnormal bleeding.**
- **8. See a doctor if you have persistent problems, such as persistent cough, persistent hoarseness, a change of bowel habits or an unexplained weight loss.**

For women:

- **9. Have a cervical smear test regularly.**
- **10. Check your breasts regularly and, if possible, undergo mammography at regular intervals over the age of 50.**

The dietary recommendations

"Frequently eat fresh fruit, vegetables and high-fibre cereals"

While evidence suggests it may be the beta-carotene, vitamin C and vitamin E in fruits, vegetables and cereals which are the active principles, it is possible that other constituents are also important. It follows that consumption of fruit and vegetables, rather than supplements, should be promoted.

Nutrients can be lost from fruit and vegetables by bad handling. You may wish to remind your patients to:

- **Ideally avoid buying damaged or bruised fruit and vegetables, but since this is often very much less expensive than perfect produce it may still be beneficial to buy and use bruised fruit rather than none at all.**
- **Select fresh or frozen rather than canned produce.**
- **Try not to peel fruit and vegetables since plant tissues in and just under the skin may contain high amounts of nutrients.**
- **Steam, stir-fry or microwave vegetables, in preference to boiling which causes higher nutrient losses.**
- **Avoid deep frying - nutrient losses are greater and the vegetables soak up the fat.**

Remember, too, that increasing consumption of high-fibre, high carbohydrate foods may help reduce fat consumption. Reducing fat consumption, though this is not yet proved, may be shown in the future to have the added benefit of helping to reduce cancer risk.

"Avoid becoming overweight and limit your intake of fatty foods"

Achievement of near-ideal body weight is desirable in relation to risk of diabetes, hypertension and cardiovascular disease as well as some cancers. Management of body weight is discussed in more detail in Chapter 2. Similarly, reduction of total fat intake is required in some people by virtue of increased risk of hypercholesterolaemia and coronary heart disease (see Chapter 3).

Fat in the diet is also discussed in Chapter 1 – A Healthy Lifestyle.

"Moderate your consumption of alcoholic drinks"

Apart from the very clear link with some cancers, moderation of alcohol is indicated in relation to hypertension (see Chapter 4), hypertriglyceridaemia (see Chapter 3) and obesity (see Chapter 2).

Supplements

The experimental evidence indicates that the dose of any one single vitamin or mineral needed to prevent cancer may sometimes be quite high. To achieve such high intakes would require the regular consumption of a vitamin supplement taken at a dose level way above the conventional recommended daily amount (RDA) – see Chapter 8. This, however, is potentially dangerous as many vitamins and minerals are toxic at high doses – this is especially so of vitamin A and selenium, to a lesser extent is so for vitamin C, and even less so for vitamin E and beta-carotene.

Summary

If patients ask about diet and the risk of cancer, the best advice to give at the present time is to follow the European Code Against Cancer, and avoid use of vitamin and mineral supplements until sound evidence justifying their use for this purpose is produced. In addition, if a patient choses to reduce salt consumption or avoid smoked, cured, pickled or barbecued foods, there seems to be no reason to counsel against this.

Chapter 7

NUTRITIONAL PROBLEMS
IN THE ELDERLY

In the UK we generally apply the term elderly to those over retirement age, ie men of 65 years and over and women of 60 years or more. This is the group in the population which is growing most rapidly. It is estimated that soon 25% of people in the UK will be over 60 and that in the ten years from 1990 to 2000 the over 80 age group, who need most care and will have most nutritional problems, will increase by 45%.

Within your practice there will be many "young elderly" who are fit and active and whose nutritional needs are not very different from the middle-aged. However, increasingly, as people survive longer there may be those who are unable or unwilling to eat properly. The requirement for GP practices to offer an annual check-up to all patients over the age of 75 may give you an opportunity to assess whether the person is able to shop for food, and is able to cook and provide an adequate diet for themselves.

There are no specific recommendations for nutrient intakes in elderly people – they are assumed to have similar needs to younger adults, except that energy requirements tend to decrease with age. Thus, to maintain an appropriate weight, energy intake will be less. A low energy intake could mean a low intake of other nutrients, so care must be taken to ensure a sensible choice of nourishing foods rather than dependence on sugary or fatty foods with few other nutrients. This means that the general guidelines for a healthy diet can apply to many elderly people, especially those young elderly who may well have another 20 years of active life ahead. However, overzealous attempts to encourage "healthy eating" in older more vulnerable groups may backfire and cause anxiety about food, disinterest in eating and inappropriate dieting. If your 85 year old patient has added sugar to tea for the last 80 odd years and had fried egg and bacon three times each week for breakfast, it is unlikely to do much harm to continue it – any damage to teeth and arteries will be well established by now.

Care should, therefore, be taken to emphasize the positive aspects of nutrition. The overall message should be to maintain an interest in and enjoyment of food which will help motivate the person to continue to cook nourishing meals and snacks even if these are simpler than in the past.

Nutritional deficiencies in the elderly

Overt signs of nutrient deficiencies in the elderly population are rare, but it is possible that, among your patients, there may be those who have subclinical nutrient deficiencies. Surveys in the UK have revealed low intakes of vitamin C, folate, riboflavin and other water soluble vitamins, vitamin D, iron, potassium, trace elements and dietary fibre in groups of elderly people both in the community and in institutions.

Various check-lists have been developed which can be used as guidelines to examine whether a particular patient might be at risk nutritionally. They look not simply at what a person eats, but also at medical and social factors which may be important (see Table 1).

Table 1. Nutritional deficiency: medical and social risk factor

Weight loss - either measured or reported
Depression - especially after bereavement
History of anorexia (poor appetite)
Poor teeth, dentures
Multiple drug therapy
Physical disability and/or mental disturbance
Arthritis in hands - difficulty in preparation of food
Evidence of alcohol abuse
Sunken eyes, inelastic skin, dry tongue may indicate dehydration

At home:
Absence of food - empty larder or fridge
Poor cooking facilities
Severely restricted mobility
Reported absence of family or good neighbours

Some of the above may be noted on a visit to the surgery, others might be reported by a health visitor or community nurse. They may result in lack of interest in food and cooking, and some of the physical factors may mean that shopping for and preparing food is difficult and simply becomes too much trouble. The elderly man whose wife has recently died is perhaps most at risk as, in many cases, the wife has always bought and cooked the food, and he may simply not know how to organize and cook his meals. In many cases, financial considerations will also be important, especially if mobility problems restrict access to cheaper shops and supermarkets.

In the DHSS report "Nutrition and Old Age" (1979)[1] it was stated that if nine or more of the risk factors identified were present then an individual was likely to be malnourished. Table 2 shows the risk factors used for this report.

Indicators of alcohol abuse were stated to be:

- **Lack of cleanliness**
- **Accidental hypothermia**
- **Hypoglycaemia**
- **Hypertriglyceridaemia**

Table 2. Social and medical risk factors	
Housebound	Living alone
No regular cooked meals	Government supplemented income
Lower social class	Depression
Chronic bronchitis	Emphysema
Difficulty in swallowing	Poor dentition
Gastrectomy	Poor mental test score
Smoking	Alcohol abuse

If the patient is dependent on alcohol, or indeed an alcoholic, then alcohol is often taken in preference to food. Appetite will also often be poor in these cases, so there is little incentive to eat.

Food habits and dietary intake

The above are factors which you may be able to observe for yourself or obtain from the medical notes; in addition, you may wish to find out something about the patient's eating habits and food intake. The following are the sort of questions which would be useful in attempting to take a diet history from an elderly patient.

(a) Can you manage to do your own shopping?

(b) If not, who does it for you?

Not being able to shop for themselves may limit the range of foods used. Being in a shop and seeing the foods available may help people to think of different meals and stimulate them into trying new foods – if someone else is doing the shopping the range of foods eaten may become quite narrow and is less likely to cover all the nutrient requirements.

(c) What foods would I find in your cupboard today?

The reply to this would give an indication as to whether the person has foods in the house which could be used in an emergency and, to some extent, whether they consider it important to make sure they have an adequate diet. A list of foods which can be suggested to be kept in store in case of bad weather or illness is shown in Table 3.

(d) Do you eat differently now you are on your own?

(e) Can you cook your favourite food?

(f) Have you lost or gained any weight recently?

(g) How often do you eat fruit, vegetables, fruit juice?

(h) Do you have milk delivered – how much do you drink each day?

(i) Does the milkman deliver other things?

Table 3. Store cupboard ideas

UHT milk in cartons (keeps for 6 months)
UHT fruit juices in cartons
Canned or packet soups
Canned meat or fish, eg corned beef, tuna, sardines, pilchards
Canned vegetables, instant potatoes. Baked beans
Canned fruits in juice, dried fruit, eg prunes, apples, apricots
Canned milk puddings and custard
Porridge oats and breakfast cereals
Crackers and biscuits
Marmalade, jam, peanut butter, bovril, marmite
Malted milk, hot chocolate. Complan or Build-Up
Stock cubes

You can also ask the patient about their day to day food intake – find out how often they eat, what sort of meals and foods they cook and the amounts of food eaten. If this questioning on diet reveals that a very limited range of foods is being eaten or that the person is having marked difficulty with food for some reason, then the help of a dietitian should be sought – she will be able to take a more detailed diet history, assess the diet and give specific advice where necessary. If patients are not eating because they are no longer able to buy or prepare their food, then it may be possible to set in motion the process of organizing a home help and/or meals on wheels. Davies[2] (1984) has identified seven risk factors which can be used to identify the elderly in need of such nutritional support – any of these could be regarded as a danger sign individually.

- **Fewer than eight main meals, hot or cold, eaten in a week.**
- **Very little milk consumed.**
- **Virtual absence of fruit and vegetables, resulting in low vitamin C intake.**
- **Wastage of food, including that supplied hot and ready to eat.**
- **Long periods in the day without food and drink.**
- **Depression or loneliness.**
- **Unexpected weight change, either a significant gain or loss.**

General advice on eating

From the questions asked above you should have some idea about your patient's eating patterns. Elderly people often prefer to have their main meal in the middle of the day and a snack in the late afternoon. If the person has a poor appetite or is unable to eat much, then it is important that the food eaten is rich in nutrients. Within the energy intake with which the patient feels comfortable and is neither gaining nor losing weight, attention should be paid to foods containing the following vitamins and minerals.

Vitamins

- B group – especially if alcohol is taken – wholegrain cereals, liver and yeast extract are major sources.

- Vitamin C – if no fresh fruit or vegetables are eaten, then it is easy to develop subclinical deficiency of this vitamin. If fruit is avoided because of poor teeth or difficulties with peeling due to arthritis, orange juice or other fruit juices fortified with vitamin C are a good substitute.

■ Vitamin D – sunlight is the major source of vitamin D – as little as 30 minutes in the sun can improve vitamin D status.

The elderly housebound can be encouraged to take fatty fish and fortified margarines. Eggs, liver and evaporated milk also contain useful amounts of the vitamin.

Minerals

■ Calcium – requirements in elderly people are similar to those for younger adults. Low calcium intake in earlier life may have left the elderly person vulnerable to fractures due to osteoporosis.

Milk and milky drinks, milky puddings, cheese and bread are everyday sources of calcium. Canned fish with bones such as sardines, pilchards and salmon are also useful.

■ Iron – lethargy and tiredness may result from a shortage of iron (and vitamin C for its absorption). Liver, red meat, corned beef and cereals fortified with iron are a good source.

■ Potassium – potassium depletion has been associated with depression, muscle weakness and mental confusion. Diets based on highly refined food with an excess of sugar may be potassium depleted. Potassium is found in all food, but especially in fruits and vegetables.

■ Magnesium – magnesium depletion follows diarrhoea or excessive losses in the urine (caused by renal diseases or osmotic diuresis), and causes apathy and muscle weakness. All foods are good sources, but cereals and vegetables are best. Gross depletion requires intravenous replacement.

General guidelines for diet for the elderly are given in the patient leaflet (see Appendix E).

Specific problems

The elderly patient who is unable to eat normal foods

If you have a patient who is unable to chew or eat normal foods and this is likely to continue for some time, it may be appropriate to consult the community dietitian who will be able to assess the situation and give advice on long term management. In the meantime, the following ideas may help and will also be useful for the patient who is temporarily unwell or unable to eat.

It is possible to maintain nutritional intake using proprietary products, such as those shown in Table 4. However, this becomes rather boring after a while and, if help is available to prepare the foods, pureeing or liquidizing ordinary foods at one or two meals per day and supplementing these with a couple of the proprietary drinks may be acceptable. The pureed foods should be made to look as appetising as possible, served separately rather than as one grey mass. Soups fortified with skim milk powder or egg, scrambled eggs, milk puddings and custard or yoghurt if liked, pureed with fruit or fruit juice, may also be acceptable.

Dietary supplements

Some elderly people may not be able to eat enough to maintain energy and nutrient requirements and, in this case, supplements such as those shown in Table 4 may be suggested to ensure that their needs are met. In other cases, you may find that it is impossible to persuade an elderly person to change from a diet which is providing sufficient energy and protein, but may be low in micronutrients. It might then be appropriate to suggest that a multivitamin supplement is prescribed.

Constipation

This is not an uncommon problem in the elderly and often results in their turning to medication for a cure. This can be avoided if they are encouraged to eat wholegrain cereal or bread regularly. (If wholemeal bread is disliked, there are some white breads fortified with fibre, eg Mighty White.) Eating pure bran should not be encouraged – flatulence, distension, bran lodging in dentures and its general unpalatability all upset the elderly.

The patient should also be encouraged to drink plenty of fluids both to soften the stools and prevent dehydration.

Table 4. Nutritional supplements

Complete nutritional supplements are available, usually as ready made milky drinks or powders to be mixed with milk or water which are then taken in place of a meal or as between meal snacks for those who simply cannot eat enough nourishing food.

These products contain energy, protein, fat, carbohydrate and a full range of vitamins and minerals.

Examples are:

Build-Up	powder mixed with milk	Nestlé
Complan	powder mixed with water or milk	Boots
Fresubin	ready to drink in carton	Fresenius
Fortimel	ready to drink in carton	Cow & Gate
Fortisip	ready to drink in carton	Cow & Gate
Fortify	powder - mix with milk	Cow & Gate

There are unflavoured, sweet flavoured and savoury versions of several of these which means that most people can find one they like

Drug-nutrient interactions

Poor nutritional status can modify drug metabolism, either increasing or decreasing the effectiveness of a drug, and some drug treatment can affect nutritional status. Elderly people may be particularly at risk because they take drugs for chronic conditions; they may be on multiple drug regimens, and their intake of nutrients may not be optimal.

Absorption of some nutrients may be impaired by drugs used commonly in the elderly population – eg anticonvulsants, cytotoxic drugs, antibiotics, cholestyramine, clofibrate, certain diuretics, liquid paraffin, anticoagulants such as phenindione, manitol, and certain anti-metabolites. Metabolism of vitamins and minerals may be altered as shown in Table 5.

Table 5. Effects of drugs on metabolism of nutrients	
Carbohydrate metabolism	Thiazides, corticosteroids, sulphonylureas, Aspirin, monoamine-oxidase inhibitors, alcohol
Lipid metabolism	Aspirin, alcohol, adrenal corticosteroids chlorpromazine phenobarbitone
Depletion of potassium	Thiazides, purgatives, adrenal steroids
Retention of water and salt	Corticosteroids, phenylbutazone, carbenoxalone
Decrease iodine uptake by thyroid gland	sulphonylureas, lithium, cobalt
Folate metabolism disturbed	Anticonvulsants, phenothiazines, tricyclic antidepressants, methotrexate
Vitamin D rendered inactive	Anticonvulsants
Vitamin C - increases excretion	Aspirin, barbiturates, corticosteroids, tetracycline
Vitamin K - synthesis by bacteria inhibited	Warfarin, antibiotics

Appetite can also be disturbed by certain drugs, eg cyclophosphamide, NSAIDS, biguanides, and the digitalis group may decrease appetite, while alcohol, thyroid hormone, steroids, insulin, sulphonylureas, and some psychotrophic drugs may increase it. Nausea, resulting in reduced food intake, may occur when such drugs as indomethacin, digoxin, theophylline and sulphonamides are taken. It is important to be aware of these possible reactions and, as new drugs come on to the market for use in conditions common in the elderly such as arthritis, diabetes and cerebrovascular disease, the practice nurse should check whether there are any known drug-nutrient interactions. The British National Formulary has up to date information on known drug-nutrient interactions. If the patient's diet is poor and unlikely to improve, it may be necessary to add supplements of the nutrients known to be affected by the particular drug.

The timing of drug-taking is also important. If a drug is more rapidly absorbed in the fasting state, the patient should understand this. Other drugs should be taken with food to minimize side-effects or increase bioavailability. It may be that a time-table for drug-taking has to be prepared for the patient.

Weight reduction

It is notoriously difficult to achieve weight reduction in the elderly and only if the weight loss is substantial will it improve mobility. Where an elderly person has been overweight for many years, it will be difficult to get them to alter their diet significantly enough to lose weight. However, by cutting out 250 Calories per day, a slow steady loss of half a pound per week (1 stone in six months) may be achieved.

Special cases

Palliative nutrition for the elderly person with cancer

It is likely that such a person has been treated as an inpatient in hospital with chemotherapy or radiotherapy and should then have been advised on how to cope with nausea, reduced appetite, changes in taste, etc. Ask if they have written instructions from the hospital and, if so, it may be useful to discuss how they can incorporate these into their own life. It is important to be sensitive to the patient's needs and circumstances. The patient may wish to try one of the "alternative" diets which have received a great deal of publicity recently, such as the Bristol diet or Gerson therapy. There are problems with these and it may be useful to contact the community dietitian for advice if the patient insists on following such a diet.

Occasionally, if the patient's appetite loss is severe, supplementary feeding via a naso-gastric tube may be necessary. Here the practice nurse and dietitian will jointly cooperate with the family. Overnight feeding is the accepted practice.

Stroke patients

Again, it is likely that the patient will have initially been rehabilitated as far as possible in hospital and will have been helped with the feeding problems. Initially, when the gag reflex was absent, the patient may have been fed by tube, but oral feeding is more likely at home. Suitable foods are those which are soft and tasty, eg thick soups and custards, yoghurt, mashed potato with egg and milk, ice creams and jellies. Many stroke patients prefer food where they can feel some texture rather than liquidized food which they cannot control and which may cause choking.

It is necessary to check periodically that the patient is managing sufficient food and, if necessary, supplements such as Complan or Build-up could be used to cover nutrient requirements.

Always remember - a little of what you fancy does you good

It is very important to get the nutrition of the elderly into perspective. The process of ageing cannot be reversed by improving vitamin status, but improved vitamin status may improve the quality of life.

1. DHSS (1979) Nutrition and health in old age. Report on Health & Social Subjects No 16. HMSO, London

2. Davies, L (1984) Nutrition and the elderly - identifying those at risk. Proc. Nutr. Soc. 295-302.

Chapter 8

VITAMINS AND MINERALS AND OTHER DIETARY SUPPLEMENTS

Vitamins and minerals are essential nutrients which we need, usually in very small amounts, to maintain health. Tables 1 and 2 respectively show the known vitamins and minerals, their role in the body and the foods from which they are obtained.

Dietary supplements

The majority of people in this country can obtain adequate amounts of vitamins and minerals from their normal diet by eating a variety of foods and supplements will rarely be needed. However, some groups of the population, such as children, pregnant and nursing mothers, and people recovering from illness, have increased requirements for certain nutrients and may occasionally be prescribed supplements temporarily. Those on very restricted therapeutic diets, which result in a limited choice of foods, may also be advised to take certain supplements all the time, but they will not be discussed in detail here as they will be receiving specialist advice.

There are also some situations where very high doses of vitamins or minerals are used as treatment for disease, eg in inborn

103

errors of metabolism, or the use of nicotinic acid in familial hyperlipidaemia. In these cases they are really being used as drugs and they will be prescribed by the doctor treating the patient, and side-effects carefully monitored.

Children

The DHSS recommends that children between the ages of 6 months and 2 years receive supplements equivalent to 200 µg vitamin A, 20 mg vitamin C and 7 µg vitamin D daily.

It is also recommended that this supplementation continue until the age of five, unless a responsible health professional is sure that the child has an appropriate energy intake from a wide range of foods.

Recently studies have been publicized suggesting that supplementing the diets of older children with vitamins and minerals improves intelligence. The original studies have been criticized and people who have tried to repeat them have not found the same beneficial effect. A recent survey of the diets of British schoolchildren suggested that their diets provided adequate nutrition, although girls tended to have low intakes of iron, calcium and riboflavin. Simply recommending a daily 300 ml of milk will satisfy the needs of the last two nutrients, and sources of iron are shown in Table 2.

Adults

People on very restricted, long-term reducing diets may benefit from a multivitamin and iron supplement. A standard 1,000–1,200 Calorie diet should however provide adequate nutrients.

There is some evidence that large doses of vitamin B6, together with evening primrose oil, may be beneficial in some women with premenstrual syndrome. Their use should ideally be medically supervised.

The elderly

Elderly housebound who are not exposed to sunlight at all may need a daily supplement of vitamin D – if their diet does not contain sufficient.

Elderly people in institutions have been shown to be at risk of B vitamin deficiency and also lack of vitamin C due to poor cooking methods. These problems may also occur in elderly people who are unable to feed themselves properly.

A daily multivitamin supplement (eg vitamins BPC) supplying amounts similar to the RDA can be advised or prescribed.

Problems with use of vitamins, minerals and other dietary supplements

There is a bewildering range of nutritional supplements available today; not simply single nutrients or combinations of nutrients, but ranges especially designed for the supposed requirements of all sorts of groups in the population. Sales of dietary supplements have trebled in the 1980's. It has been estimated that 20% of the population regularly takes a dietary supplement and their sale is providing lucrative business for the increasing number of health food shops, chemists and supermarkets who stock them. Currently vitamins and minerals are sold under food laws in the UK and Europe, but it is likely that the EEC will reclassify these as medicines and that from 1992 there will be much more stringent controls over their sale. At present there is little advice about supplementation available from qualified health professionals and people are unaware of the potential hazards of taking too much of a supplement or of the possible interactions with other nutrients.

Vitamin and mineral supplements are often taken in large doses, in amounts much higher than the RDA, and health care workers are concerned about the potential effects of overdoses (see Table 3). This is most likely to be a problem with fat soluble vitamins, such as vitamin A or D, because these are stored in the liver, but excess of many other nutrients can be harmful in certain situations. Nutrients interact with each other in the body and supplements can cause a dietary imbalance which may affect the rate of absorption, excretion and requirement of other vitamins, minerals, proteins, fats and carbohydrates. If the person is apparently healthy and eating a well balanced diet, it is perhaps better not to upset nutritional status by taking supplements.

If for any reason supplements are deemed necessary, the following advice should be given:

- **Follow the prescription or manufacturer's instructions about dose.**
- **Never take any vitamins or minerals in excess - a lot is not necessarily better than a little.**
- **Remember to check the ingredients if the patient is on a special therapeutic diet - supplements may contain sugars, colourings, or flavourings.**
- **Always keep supplements out of the reach of children.**

Nutritional supplements

Apart from the vitamin and mineral supplements which may be used if a person is at risk of developing a deficiency of particular nutrients, there are other supplements which may be useful in cases where a patient is unable to take a full range of foods. Nutritional supplements are considered in Table 4 of Chapter 7.

It is best not to use them as the only source of nutrition for longer than a day or two – if you have a patient who can not eat ordinary food for any reason, it is best to discuss the problem with a dietitian.

Table 1. Vitamins :
Sources, functions and deficiencies

Vitamin	Function	Sources	Possible Deficiency
FAT SOLUBLE			
A (Retinol)	Keeps mucus membranes healthy. Essential for vision in dim light.	Dairy products, eggs, enriched margarine, cod liver oil.	Night blindness (rare - sometimes seen in alcoholics
Beta-carotene	Antioxidant properties - "free radical" scavenger	Deep green and orange vegetables - carotene converted to retinol in the body.	It is now suggested that adequate intake may protect against some cancers.
D	Necessary for bone formation. Regulates calcium metabolism.	Fish liver oils, fatty fish, eggs, enriched margarine, butter. Most important: made in body when skin exposed to sunlight.	Rickets, osteomalacia. Rare in Caucasians. May be seen in Asian children, adolescents and women. Elderly housebound may have poor dietary intake and no exposure to sunshine.
E	Possibly antioxidant - protects cells from free radical damage.	Vegetable oils, eggs, butter, wholegrain cereals, wheatgerm.	Extremely rare.
K	Blood clotting, involved in energy metabolism.	Green leafy vegetables, fruit, nuts, wholegrain cereals.	Prolonged clotting time. Bleeding tendency. May be seen in diseases where malabsorption occurs, eg cystic fibrosis, liver disease. Broad spectrum antibiotics destroy the gut flora which make vitamin K.

Vitamin	Function	Sources	Possible Deficiency
WATER SOLUBLE			
Thiamin (B1)	Energy metabolism especially carbohydrate.	Wholegrain cereals, seeds, nuts, pulses, meat - especially offal.	Unlikely in normal circumstances. Deficiency of this and other B vitamins sometimes seen in alcoholics.
Riboflavin (B2)	Energy metabolism especially protein and fat.	Milk and milk products, meat, liver, eggs, yeast extract.	Angular stomatitis, sore tongue, lips. Has been seen in elderly on very restricted diets.
Niacin	Energy metabolism.	Meat especially offal, pulses, nuts, yeast extract, fortified cereals.	Unlikely to be seen in normal circumstances.
Pyridoxine (B6)	Protein metabolism. Blood formation. Health of nervous system.	Meat especially offal, fish, poultry, yeast, wholegrain cereals.	Rare, but some drugs may cause deficiency, eg Isoniazid, contraceptive pills containing oestrogen.
Folate	Formation of all cells in body. Red blood cell formation. Health of nervous system.	Liver, pulses, wholegrain cereals, green vegetables.	Megaloblastic anaemia. May occur in toddlers, people with very restricted diets. May prevent neural tube defects in pregnancy, so is needed preconceptually.
Cyanocobalamin (B12)	Red blood cell formation. Formation of all cells. Important for health of nervous system.	Meat, fish, milk and milk products.	May occur in strict vegans who eat no animal products. Occurs in atrophic gastritis (pernicious anaemia).
Biotin	Protein and fat metabolism.	Offal, pulses, yeast extract, nuts, green vegetables.	Unlikely.

Vitamin	Function	Sources	Possible Deficiency
Pantothenic acid	All metabolism.	All foods but especially liver, egg yolk, yeast, vegetables.	Unlikely.
Ascorbic acid (C)	Maintenance of all tissues especially connective tissue. Essential for healing.	Citrus fruit and berries, potatoes, vegetables, tomatoes.	Scurvy. Unlikely, but sub-clinical deficiencies may occur. Elderly with diet low in fruit and vegetables, and anywhere where vegetables are overcooked.

Table 2. Minerals and trace elements: Sources, functions and deficiencies

Mineral	Function	Sources	Possible Deficiency
Calcium	Formation and maintenance of bones and teeth. Blood clotting, nerve and muscle function.	Milk, cheese, bread, tinned fish - tuna, sardines, salmon, pulses, nuts, hard water.	Acceleration of osteoporosis - low calcium intake & low exercise when young may result in less dense bones when older. Adequate intake may slow rate at which bone is lost.
Iron	Formation of red blood cells. Many roles in metabolism.	Offal, red meat, corned beef, pulses, wholegrain cereals, oats and enriched breakfast cereals, green vegetables, dried fruit, vitamin C aids absorption.	Iron deficiency anaemia. Look out for this in premenopausal women, possibly in adolescents and children. Slimmers and those following low fat diets may have low intake. In pregnancy anaemia may be suspected because of dilution of blood - only supplement if anaemia definitely present.

Mineral	Function	Sources	Possible Deficiency
Zinc	Tissue repair, growth and development, bone metabolism, smell and taste mechanism.	Offal, meat, shellfish, egg, cheese, wholegrain cereals.	Possibly small stature. Hair loss, skin rashes, poor healing, impaired taste acuity. Supplements may help heal skin ulcers.
Copper	Coenzyme for many enzymes including iron absorption. Formation of bone. Growth. Immune system.	Green vegetables, fish, oysters, liver, pulses, dried fruit.	Rare.
Magnesium	Energy metabolism.	Most foods, but especially cereals and vegetables.	Losses usually in urine or faeces, causing apathy and muscle weakness. After diarrhoea and osmotic diuresis.
Selenium	Acts with vitamin E to prevent free radical damage.	English wheat, mushrooms, brazil nuts, meat, offal, eggs, milk.	Cardiomyopathy and osteopathy, seen in long-term TPN. Low serum levels may be associated with increased risk of some cancers and CHD.
Chromium	Carbohydrate and lipid metabolism.	Offal, brewer's yeast, nuts, wholegrains.	May predispose to maturity onset DM.

Recommended dietary allowances (RDAs)

Recommended dietary allowances are the amounts of energy and nutrients recommended to cover the needs of groups of healthy people. They are not intended to be used for individuals, but in practice they are a useful guideline.

In some cases, there is no RDA because there is insufficient information about requirements. The USA "safe and adequate" intake gives an estimate of a suitable range of intakes.

Table 3. Some common dietary supplements: Beneficial effects, possible side-effects, and RDA

Supple-ment	Possible uses	Common misconceptions corrected	Toxic effects	RDA
Vitamin A and beta-carotene	Supplements may be given in trials to study possible cancer preventing effects especially of beta-carotene.		Retinol - headache, drowsiness, skin changes, anorexia, weight loss, muscle pain, chronic liver disease.	750 µg(Retinol equivalents)
Vitamin D	May be given to the elderly housebound, and children during winter months. (Pregnant Asian women may be given supplements of A & D as well as iron and folate.)		Hypercalcaemia in infants, hypercalaemia and metastatic calcification, renal stones, hypercholesterolaemia, hypertension.	10 µg (7µg children under 5)
Vitamin C	Elderly living alone or in institutions with poor dietary intake.	No evidence for prevention of common cold but may reduce severity of symptoms (50-100 mg/d). No effect in reducing serum cholesterol.	Kidney stones because of increased excretion of water and oxalate. Breakdown of RBC. Impairment of white cell function (doses over 2 g/d). Decreased B12 and increased iron absorption.	30 mg
Vitamin E		No evidence for beneficial effects on ageing, sterility, diabetes, skin disorders, or muscular dystrophy.	Prolongs clotting time by antagonizing vitamin K. Increases anti-coagulant effect of Warfarin.	No UK RDA: USA 8-10 mg

Supplement	Possible uses	Common misconceptions corrected	Toxic effects	RDA
Nicotinic Acid	Given as a drug to reduce plasma lipids.		Histamine release, flushing, aggravation of asthma (100 mg). Hyperglycaemia. Aggravation of DM and peptic ulcer. Hepatotoxic and may cause jaundice. Gouty arthritis incidence increased.	15-18 mg
Vitamin B6	Given with Isoniazid treatment. May benefit nausea in pregnancy. May help prevent recurrence of breast cancer.	No conclusive evidence for beneficial effects in PMT, postnatal depression. No evidence for improved sports performance.	Peripheral neuropathy. Antagonizes Levodopa, penicillamine and phenytoin. Dependency in adults and infants of women taking large doses in pregnancy.	No UK RDA: USA 1.6-2.0 mg
Folate	May prevent neural tube defects in women already having one NTD child. Megaloblastic anaemia due to folate deficiency.		Insomnia, irritability, masking of B12 deficiency. Antagonizes phenytoin.	No UK RDA: USA 180-200µg
B Vitamins	May be advised if taking antibiotics.	No evidence for improvement of sports performance.	As for individual vitamins.	
ABIDEC Children's vitamin drops	Children up to the age of 2 and up to 5 if poor appetite.		As for individual vitamins	Do not exceed stated dose.
EFAMOL (evening primrose oil)	May benefit PMT, eczema.			

Supplement	Possible uses	Common misconceptions corrected	Toxic effects	RDA
Fish Oils (eg MAXE-PA, cod liver oil)	Reduces plasma triglycerides. May help prevent secondary myocardial infarction.	Evidence for prevention of CHD not conclusive.	Prolonged clotting time.	
Multivitamins (with/without iron)	Slimmers, elderly with poor appetite.		Unlikely if taken in prescribed quantity. Iron may cause constipation.	
Iron	Iron deficiency anaemia.	Not necessary in pregnancy unless proven anaemic.	Unlikely if taken in prescribed quantity. Iron may cause constipation.	10-12 mg
Calcium	Necessary if very low dietary intake for any reason, especially in children.	Does not prevent osteoporosis, but adequate intake may delay it.	Large doses may cause kidney stones.	500 mg
Selenium	May protect against CHD and certain cancers. Some suggest use if low levels in soil. Benefits not proven.		Hair loss, nail changes, peripheral neuropathy, disorders of the nervous system.	No UK RDA: USA RDA 55-70 µg/d
Selenium ACE		Common supplement - selenium plus anti-oxidant vitamins - suggested to prevent cancers. Not proven.		
Zinc	Patients with leg ulcers.	Not proven to be beneficial preconceptually or in pregnancy. Not proven to protect against or improve symptoms of common cold.	Metallic taste in mouth, nausea.	No UK RDA: USA 12-15 mg/d

Supple-ment	Possible uses	Common misconceptions corrected	Toxic effects	RDA
Chromium	"Hypoglycaemia". Benefits not proven.	No evidence of benefi-cial effects in CHD.		No RDA*

* "Safe & Adequate" 50-200 µg/d

NB: RDA's are given for adults. Figures for men and women are sometimes different, and requirements for children are usually lower. See original sources listed in Appendix 5.

Chapter 9

PROBLEMS OF MOTIVATION AND COMPLIANCE

Food is a basic need in life. Some people will attach great importance to it and others will be much more pragmatic. But as soon as changes are made to what we eat, the amount we eat and how we cook it, food and diet take up a bigger proportion of our time and thoughts. A diet then becomes food that gives not the pleasure it did before, but food that is a chore imposed upon us for the sake of our health.

The dietary advice which will be given by practice nurses will mean long term changes in both the lifestyle and food habits of the patients and their families, to a varying degree. A person's ability to implement and maintain dietary changes will depend on their personality, whether they live alone or in a family, their role within that family, who does the shopping and cooking, whether they work and the "food culture" at work. Factors that can influence compliance will depend on perceived effectiveness of the diet, ie does it "work", and the ease with which dietary changes can be incorporated into a patient's daily routine.

A therapeutic diet is given to treat a specific condition and these diets will range from the relatively basic and common low energy diets for obesity to extensive prohibition of foods as in food allergy/intolerance. To help anyone with a dietary problem it is important to familiarize yourself with the diet sheets they are using. If your practice uses diet sheets supplied by the health authority dietetic department, make sure you have copies and you know what advice they are giving.

Some common problems

The most common problems with patients trying to follow a specific diet are:

- **The diet is "not working" (usually low energy diets for weight reduction).**
- **The cost is too high.**
- **Not liking the foods recommended on the diet.**
- **Women may find it difficult to follow the diet and feed other members of the family.**
- **Unsupportive family and friends.**
- **Eating out, holidays, special occasions.**

"Your diet doesn't work"

A patient's ability to follow the advice will depend on their motivation and ability to eat the foods recommended. Diets themselves do not "work" or "not work"; it is the patient's ability to restrict their intake, or change the kinds of foods they eat or their cooking methods, which brings them success or failure. Diets "work" the closer the patient can keep to the advice given but, quite reasonably, no one should expect patients to do this for a hundred per cent of the time. Compliance may be improved by suggesting that the patient follows the diet closely for weekdays, but is more lenient at weekends, or follows the diet strictly for two weeks and then has a week off the diet. The usual objection to these sorts of changes is that patients feel their weight will increase should they stop the diet. It should be pointed out to them that this increase in weight is probably due to water retention, should be only about 1 kg, and will probably be lost once the diet is restarted. On their days off the diet, they should be sensible about what they eat and not indulge in all the foods they have been advised not to eat, eg cakes, sweets, chocolate, fried foods, alcohol. They should also not weigh themselves on a Monday after a weekend off the diet, but leave it until Friday after five days of more rigid dieting.

"Lettuce is for rabbits"

Problems occur with the acceptability of the actual foods recommended. The common areas of dislike are:

- Salad on a reducing diet.
- Low fat spreads and skimmed milk.
- Small quantities of red meat.
- No hard cheeses on a lipid lowering diet.

For some reason, people think that salad has some magical property that will make them lose weight and so they must eat it as part of their energy controlled diet. It is one of the myths of losing weight. Many people, especially men, do not enjoy salad as part of every main meal and vegetables are an acceptable alternative, including vegetables such as peas and baked beans. Baked beans on wholemeal toast or in a jacket potato are very acceptable meals for both low fat and reducing diets.

Low fat spreads, because of their composition, contain a lot of water which alters their consistency and taste, making them very different from butter and margarine. If, after persevering and trying various brands of low fat spreads, the patient still finds them unacceptable, then there are two alternatives you might suggest.

The patient could use butter or, preferably, a polyunsaturated margarine, but in small quantities. As a guide, a 250g packet or carton should last one person about two weeks. Alternatively, they could look for something else to spread on their bread – sandwiches can often be made without fat if the filling is soft, preserves can be spread on toast in place of fat or cheese, or yeast extract might be acceptable. These contain less than half the energy value of butter or margarine and less energy than low fat spreads.

117

Many people find skimmed milk unacceptable when they have been used to full cream silver top milk. Semi-skimmed milk is a suitable alternative, particularly for cereals and puddings.

Some patients will be used to eating red meat each day. The dietary advice for hyperlipidaemia and general healthy eating advice suggest that red meat should be reduced to about three meals per week. Finding acceptable alternatives can be difficult, the usual ones being fish, poultry and other protein sources such as cereals and pulses.

Although it can be difficult to get people who do not eat pulses as a regular part of their diet to start eating them, there are two beans that are already a part of many diets – baked beans and red kidney beans (in chilli con carne). The use of these foods can be extended from beans on toast or as a vegetable to using them as a filling for a jacket potato or with pasta in, for example, the meat layer in lasagne. Red kidney beans, or any other beans, can be used in dishes that are based on meat – stews and casseroles – to take the place of perhaps half of the meat.

Using more fish should be encouraged. Lunchtime sandwiches could be filled with tuna, mackerel or sardines (tinned in brine not oil) instead of cheese. Main meals such as fish pie or fish cakes or simply fish baked in the oven could be suggested.

For lovers of hard cheeses a diet that substitutes alternatives which do not have the same flavour can be difficult to follow. One solution is to have a hard cheese occasionally, but in reduced quantity. This can be achieved by grating or slicing in thin slices with a cheese parer.

"I can't afford it"

For some patients cost can be a problem: they might not have enough money, some foods you are asking the patients to eat cost more, or they might think that they have to buy special diet foods. If dietary habits are changing, then the money saved on buying cakes, biscuits and sweets could be spent on other foods such as fruit or more vegetables. If patients have limited resources they may be advised to purchase cheaper supermarket own-brands of foods where available. Vegetables and fruit are often cheaper in the market or from street barrows than in shops and supermarkets, and shopping later in the day, close to supermarket closing time, can often realize bargains in bread, fruits and dairy produce.

There is no need to buy special foods or special meals as they are expensive. Similar meals can be prepared at home which the rest of the family can also eat. Sauces for spaghetti can be kept low in energy by not frying any of the ingredients, but putting them all into a pan together with stock or water and tinned tomatoes and boiling till cooked. A similar method can also be used to stew meat.

"There's only me on a diet"

It is important to remember that the healthy eating recommendations are perfectly suitable for the majority of the family. However, there will be situations where some family members will require, for example, more energy than the dieter. In this case there has to be some compromise – the family can add fat to their jacket potatoes or may have chips with their meal or a different pudding, while the basis of the meal is the same. This calls for the dieter to be strict with themselves, which is not easy, but they should be reminded of their goal and supported in their efforts.

"Just one won't hurt you"

Other family members and often friends may be unsupportive of the dieter, who will need their support and also the support of the person who does the shopping and/or cooking. If this person has not been at the original consultation, then they may not understand what is involved. This can be remedied by seeing the dieter and the cook together and going through the diet with both of them. If it is the cook who is on the diet and the rest of the family are unsupportive, this is more difficult to remedy and the cook will have to learn to ignore the family.

If someone is trying to lose weight, having been unsuccessful in the past, then the family may ridicule the current attempt,

119

especially if smaller portions are served or different meals eaten. It will be helpful if the dieter eats meals similar to the rest of the family but is careful about how they are cooked. For example, traditional Sunday lunch could be a couple of slices of lean meat, 1–2 small roast potatoes, plenty of vegetables, small Yorkshire pudding and some gravy with fresh fruit or fruit tinned in natural juice for pudding.

Friends who press people to eat or drink foods they are trying to avoid can be a nuisance. There is no easy solution to this problem; it can be dealt with only by a polite refusal.

Situations such as socializing in a pub can be helped by drinking smaller quantities, eg half-pints instead of pints, making drinks last longer or changing the type of drink. There are now many low alcohol and alcohol-free drinks available, but it must be remembered that they are not energy-free. If a patient wishes to drink alcohol, then a spirit diluted with a low calorie mixer might be suitable. This contains about one-third of the energy of a pint of beer, but obviously cannot be drunk freely!

People who work in an office environment may have to cope with the ubiquitous birthday or leaving celebration which always seems to include a high energy/high fat cake. This sort of thing must be put into perspective – where it happens rarely then it should be eaten without the dieter feeling guilty. Food does fill an important social function and this must not be taken away from the dieter.

Special occasions

Eating out, holidays, special occasions, all seem to provide excuses for not following dietary advice. As they are fairly regular occurrences then patients need advice on how to cope with them, enjoy themselves and remain reasonably close to their diet. It is the frequency with which they occur that presents the long term problem. Eating food and cakes provided at a wedding reception or special family occasion will make no difference to the effectiveness of most diets. The patient should follow their diet up to the event, eat sensibly at the occasion and continue with their diet at the next meal. It is not always a good idea to miss meals on the special day as this will make them feel extra hungry and any good intentions will disappear. Special occasions should not be used as excuses for abandoning a diet as it is probably only one meal in a week of twenty other meals: keeping to dietary advice under adverse conditions is part of lifestyle changes with which the patient has to come to terms.

Holidays can be a problem depending on where they are spent. Many hotels will cater for special diets and airlines will provide special meals if booked in advance. Self-catering holidays are ideal as the dieter can cope as if at home. Foreign holidays may be more difficult if the place, language and foods are very different from those with which the patient is familiar. If travelling with a holiday company, then the company's resort representative should be able to help either with meals in the hotel or with guidance to local dishes. If the patient has made their own arrangements then dietary requirements may be misunderstood because of the language barrier. Guide books will give some help on local dishes.

"It doesn't fit in with my work - I eat out a lot"

People who have jobs which involve a lot of entertaining or eating out in pubs or restaurants, may find some dietary restrictions difficult to follow. The most helpful way to deal with this is to go through an imaginary menu with the patient, discussing what may be suitable choices and what should be avoided. First course could consist of fruit juice, fruit cocktail, melon or fish, with no fried foods or dishes in sauce chosen. For the main course, chicken or fish, a grill or maybe the vegetarian option, provided it is not cheese-based or in a sauce, are all suitable. Salad or vegetables without dressings or sauces are fine as are potatoes without added fat, such as boiled or jacket. The sweet course may be omitted or there may be fresh fruit or fruit salad – no cream. A glass of dry white wine could be included with the meal if necessary.

Solving problems arising from trying to adhere to a diet takes commonsense, patience, a sense of humour and a little knowledge of food and nutrition. Some patients will cope with the changes their diet imposes well, others will not. These patients may decide that the lifestyle changes are not acceptable, even for the sake of their health. However, they may be able to make some small changes, such as using a lower fat milk or a low fat spread, or changing the type of bread they eat. Indeed, for some patients these small changes may be the best way of beginning and, with encouragement and time, they may be able to make more drastic changes. The patient has to make the ultimate decision as to whether the dietary changes are acceptable and even beneficial. The role of the practice nurse is the same as that of the dietitian – to advise, encourage and support.

Appendix 1

DIETARY GUIDELINES

| DIETARY COMPO-NENT | CURRENT ESTI-MATED INTAKE | NACNE PROPOSALS | | COMA RECOMMENDA-TIONS |
		SHORT TERM	LONG TERM	
Energy in-take		Recommend adjustment to the types of food eaten and an increased exercise programme so that adult body weight is achieved and/or maintained within the optimal limits of weight-for-height		
Total fat intake	42% of total energy	34% of total energy	30% of total energy	35% of total energy
Saturated fat intake	20% of total energy	15% of total energy	10% of total energy	15% of total energy
Polyunsatu-rated fat in-take	5% of total energy. P:S ratio 0.23	No specific recommendation.		Recommend that the P:S ratio be in-creased to approx. 0.45.
Cholesterol intake	350-450 mg/d	No specific recommendation.		
Sucrose in-take	38 kg/head/year	34 kg/head/year	20 kg/head/year	The intake of simple sugars should not be increased.
Fibre intake	20 g/head/day	25 g/head/day	30 g/head/day	No specific recom-mendation.

123

DIETARY COMPONENT	CURRENT ESTIMATED INTAKE	NACNE PROPOSALS		COMA RECOMMENDATIONS
		SHORT TERM	LONG TERM	
Salt intake	8-12 g/head/day	1 g/head/day reduction	3 g/head/day reduction	Salt intake should not be increased. Ways should be sought to decrease the intake. The amount added in and after cooking should be decreased immediately.
Alcohol intake	4-9% of total energy	5% of total energy	4% of total energy	Excessive intake should be avoided on general health grounds.
Protein intake	11% of total	No recommendation.		No specific recommendation, but highlighting that animal protein tends to be associated with saturated fatty acids and vegetable protein with dietary fibre.

Appendix 2

HIGH FIBRE FOODS

Wholemeal or high-bran breads. Fortified white breads.

Wholegrain or bran-enriched cereals, eg porridge oats, All-Bran, Branflakes, Weetabix, Shredded Wheat, muesli.

Wholemeal pasta and brown rice. Other whole cereals, eg bulghar wheat, oats, barley.

Biscuits, cakes, puddings and pastry made with wholemeal flour, oats, dried fruit and nuts, eg fruit cake, digestive biscuits, bran biscuits, crispbreads.

Vegetables of all kinds especially peas, beans and lentils. Potatoes are best eaten with the skin.

Dried fruit, eg apricots, sultanas, prunes. Fruits of all kinds contribute some fibre to the diet especially if eaten with the skin on.

Nuts (not whole for under fives).

Appendix 3

DIETARY RULES OF MINORITY GROUPS

The three main Asian religious groups - Hindus, Muslims and Sikhs – each have food restrictions.

Hindus

1. May not eat meat of any kind. If less strict, may eat lamb, chicken, or white fish, but unlikely to eat beef or pork.

2. Very strict Hindus may not eat eggs.

3. Fats, such as dripping, margarine and lard, are not allowed. Ghee and vegetable oil are used in cooking.

4. Strict Hindus will be unwilling to eat food unless they are sure that it has not been cooked in utensils which have been in contact with meat or fish.

Sikhs

This began as an offshoot of Hinduism, but food is a matter for each individual's conscience and they are often not as strict as Hindus. Some, especially women, are vegetarian, but many eat lamb, chicken and fish.

Alcohol is forbidden, but some men do take alcoholic drinks.

Muslims

All foods are lawful (Halal), except the following:

1. Foods from the pig or any carnivorous animal.

2. Meat which has not been ritually slaughtered (Kosher meat may be acceptable).

3. Alcohol in any form.

A devout Muslim may refuse food if he can't be sure it doesn't contain an unlawful food or that it has not been in contact with such a food.

Jews

The following rules are part of the discipline and way of life of the Jewish religion.

1. No pork or pork products.

2. Meat of animals with a cloven hoof which chew the cud are allowed, eg deer, goat, cattle, sheep.

3. No birds of prey. Chicken, turkey, duck, goose, partridge, pheasant, and pigeon are allowed.

4. Fish with fins and scales are allowed. No shellfish.

5. Meat and milk must not be served at the same meal or cooked together. 6. Animals and birds are slaughtered by the ritual method – meat is then described as Kosher.

Appendix 4

CALORIE CHART

Bacon:	back, grilled	2 rashers (1.5 oz)	162
	fried	2 rashers (1.5 oz)	186
	streaky, grilled	3 rashers (1 oz)	126
Beef:	roast topside	4 slices (4 oz)	256
	stew	1 ladle (6 oz)	202
Butter:		For 1 slice of bread ($\frac{1}{4}$ oz)	51
Cheese:	Cheddar	Matchbox cube (1 oz)	121
	Camembert type	Matchbox cube (1 oz)	90
	Edam	Matchbox cube (1 oz)	91
Chicken:	breast, roast	No skin (4 oz)	184
Cod:	fillet, grilled	(6 oz)	166
	in batter	(8 oz)	447
Corned beef:		2 slices (2.5 oz)	172
Cream:	double	1 tablespoon	89
	single	1 tablespoon	42
Egg:	boiled/poached	1 size 2 egg	95
	fried	1 size 2 egg	127
Fish:	cakes, fried	2	188
	fingers, fried	4	209
Gammon:	grilled	7 oz raw weight	342

Ham:		2 thin slices (2 oz)	60
Hot dog sausage:		3	180
Kipper:	grilled fillet	1 (approx 4 oz)	229
Lamb chop:	grilled, lean	Approx 3 oz	188
	roast leg incl. fat	2 slices (approx 4 oz)	319
Lasagne:		Half a plateful (approx 10 oz)	453
Low fat spread:		For 1 slice bread (1/4 oz)	25
Luncheon meat:		3 slices (2 oz)	175
Macaroni cheese:		Approx 7 oz	374
Margarine:	Hard/soft/polyunsaturated	For 1 slice bread (1/4 oz)	51
Milk:	condensed	Approx 1 oz	80
	evaporated	1 tablespoon	31
	fresh, silver top	1/2 pint	182
	semi-skimmed	1/2 pint	126
	skimmed	1/2 pint	92
Plaice:	in breadcrumbs, fried	1 fillet (approx 6 oz)	410
Pork chop:	grilled	Approx 5 oz	305
Pork pie:		1 individual (5 oz)	545
Prawns:		Approx 1 oz	26
Quiche:		1/6th whole quiche (2.5 oz)	273
Salami:		4 slices (2 oz)	275
Salmon:	tinned	Approx 3.5 oz	162
Sausages:	pork, grilled	3 large	400
	beef, grilled	3 large	333
Sausage roll:		1 (2 oz)	277
Scotch egg:		1 (4 oz)	312

Shepherd's pie:		2 tablespoons	208
Spaghetti bolognese:		Approx 8 oz	287
Steak:	rump, grilled	8 oz raw weight	218
Yoghurt:	fruit, low fat	1 carton	142
	plaion, low fat	1 carton	78
Apple, orange, pear, peach:		1	46
Banana:		1 medium (4 oz, no skin)	94
Baked beans:		8 oz	144
Biscuits:	half-coated chocolate digestives	2	146
	plain digestives	2	141
	cream, sandwich	2	123
	plain, eg rich tea	2	73
Bread:	wholemeal	1 medium slice from large loaf	86
	white	1 medium slice from large loaf	94
Cream crackers:		2	61
Crispbreads:		3	80

Appendix 5

FURTHER READING

General

Committee on Diet and Health (Food & Nutrition Board, National Research Council). Diet and Health: Implications for reducing Chronic Disease Risk. Washington, DC: National Academy Press 1980.

Thomas B, Ed. Manual of Dietetic Practice. Oxford: Blackwell Scientific Publications 1988.

Passmore R & Eastwood MA, Eds. Human Nutrition and Dietetics. Eighth Edition. Edinburgh: Churchill Livingstone, 1986.

Westland P. The High-Fibre Cookbook - Recipes for good health. London: Martin Dunitz 1982.

Open University. The Open University guide to healthy eating. London: Rambletree Publishing Ltd 1985.

Obesity

Garrow JS. Treat Obesity seriously - a clinical manual. Edinburgh: Churchill Livingstone, 1981.

Garrow JS. Obesity and related disease. 2nd Edn. Edinburgh: Churchill Livingstone, 1988.

Coronary Heart Disease & High Blood Cholesterol

Lewis B, Assmann G, Mancini M, Stein Y, Eds. Handbook of Coronary Heart Disease Prevention. London: Current Medical Literature Ltd. 1989.

Thompson GR. A Handbook of Hyperlipidaemia. London: Current Science Ltd. 1989.

Hypertension

MacGregor G. The salt free diet book. New York: Arco Publishing 1985.

Diabetes Mellitus

Day JL. The Diabetes Handbook: Non-Insulin dependent Diabetes. Wellingborough: Thorsons (in association with the British Diabetic Association) 1986.

Day JL. The Diabetes Handbook: Insulin dependent Diabetes. Wellingborough: Thorsons (in association with the British Diabetic Association) 1986.

Metcalfe J. Better Cookery for Diabetics. London: British Diabetic Association 1985.

Metcalfe J. Cooking the new diabetic way. London: British Diabetic Association 1987.

Diet and the risk of Cancer

Bingham S. Diet and Cancer (a briefing paper). London: Health Education Authority 1990.

Nutritional problems in the Elderly

Davies L. Easy cooking for one or two. Harmondsworth: Penguin 1972.

Vitamins and Minerals

Committee on Medical Aspects of Food Policy. Recommended daily amounts of Food Energy and Nutrients for groups of people in the United Kingdom. Report on Health and Social Subjects No 15, Department of Health and Social Security. London: HMSO 1979.

Subcommittee on the tenth edition of the RDAs (of the Food and Nutrition Board, National Research Council). Recommended Dietary Allowances. 10th Edition. Washington, DC: National Academy Press 1989.

Appendix 6

SOME USEFUL ADDRESSES

Beecham Products, Beecham House, Great West Road, Brentford, Middlesex TW8 9BD. Tel: 081-560 5151

Boots Company plc, 1 Thane Road West, Nottingham NG2 3AA. Tel: Nottingham 56111

British Diabetic Association, 10 Queen Anne Street, London W1M 0BD. Tel: 071-323 1531

British Dietetic Association, Daimler House, Paradise Circus, Queensway, Birmingham B1 2BJ. Tel: 021-643 5483

British Heart Foundation, 102 Gloucester Road, London W1. Tel: 071-935 0185

British Nutrition Foundation, 15 Belgrave Square, London SW1X 8PS. Tel: 071-235 4904

Butter Information Council Ltd, Tubs Hill House, London Road, Sevenoaks, Kent TN13 1BL. Tel: 0732-460060

Chest, Heart and Stroke Association, Tavistock House, North Tavistock Square, London W1L 9JE. Tel: 071-387 3012/3/4

Coeliac Society, PO Box 220, High Wycombe, Bucks HP11 2HY. Tel: 0494-37278

Coronary Prevention Group, 60 Great Ormond Street, London WC1. Tel: 071-833 3687

Cow and Gate Ltd, Cow and Gate House, Trowbridge, Wilts BA14 8YX. Tel: Trowbridge 68381

Family Heart Association, 9 West Way, Botley, Oxford OX2 0JB. Tel: 0865 798969

Flour Advisory Bureau, 21 Arlington Street, London SW1. Tel: 071-493 2521/6786

The Flora Project for Heart Disease Prevention, 24-28 Bloomsbury Way, London WC1A 2PX. Tel: 071-242 0936

Food and Drink Federation, 6 Catherine Street, London WC2B 5JJ. Tel:071-836 2460

Fruit Information Services Ltd, E204, Fruit and Vegetable Market, New Covent Garden Market, London SW8. Tel: 071-720 7486

Health Visitors Association, 50 Southwark Street, London SE1 1UN. Tel: 071-378 7255

Meat and Livestock Commission, PO Box 44, Queensway House, Bletchley. Tel: Milton Keynes 74941

Milk Marketing Board, Thames Ditton, Surrey KT7 0EL. Tel: 081- 398 4101

National Dairy Council, 5 John Princes Street, London W1M 0AP. Tel: 071-499 7822

Nestle Company Ltd, Health Care Division, St. Georges House, Croydon, Surrey CR9 1NR. Tel: 081-686 3333

Nutrasweet Information Centre, 59 Russell Square, London W1. Tel: 071-636 9068

Nutrition Society, 10 Cambridge Court, 210 Shepherd's Bush Road, London W6 7NJ. Tel: 071-602 0228

Nutrition and Dietetic Consultants, 97 Harley Street, London W1N 4DF. Tel: 071-487 3740

Potato Marketing Board, 50 Hans Crescent, London SW1X 0NB. Tel: 071-589 4874

The Quaker Oats Nutrition Centre, 24-28 Bloomsbury Way, London WC1A 2PX. Tel: 071-831 6262

Royal College of Nursing, 20 Cavendish Square, London W1. Tel: 071-409 3333

Scotia Pharmaceuticals Ltd, Woodbridge Meadows, Guildford, Surrey GU1 1BA. Tel: 0483-574949

The Sugar Bureau, Duncan House, Dolphin Square, London SW1. Tel: 071-828 9465

The Vegetarian Society, 53 Marloes Road, London W8. Tel: 071- 937 7739/1714

Patient Information Leaflets

Nutrition Matters

A HEALTHY DIET

It is now thought that in countries such as the UK many serious disorders are caused at least partly by eating too much food or choosing the wrong types of food. Because many of us eat too much fat and sugar and not enough dietary fibre we are likely to be overweight and diseases such as heart disease, high blood pressure and cancers are common. Certain changes in our diet may prevent many of these diseases. The changes recommended are:

● Increase the amount of starchy foods and dietary fibre
● Reduce the amount of fat eaten
● Eat less sugar
● Eat less salt
● Limit alcohol intake.

Following the guidelines below will ensure that you get enough of the nutrients essential for health – proteins, vitamins and minerals. The best way of doing this is to eat a variety of foods as part of a regular pattern of meals.

A healthy diet does not mean that you must avoid all food treats. As long as the day-to-day diet is sensible, the occasional chunk of cream cake, rich restaurant meal, or bar of chocolate won't be a problem.

THE BASIS OF A

HEALTHY DIET

Foods which are rich in starch and dietary fibre should be the mainstay of your diet. Our ancestors thought in terms of bread and cheese, potatoes and meat rather than meat and potatoes, cheese and bread, and ideally we should start to think in the same way.

EAT MOST OF:

● Bread especially wholemeal bread (if you don't like wholemeal, eat more white bread or use those fortified with fibre)
● Wholegrain breakfast cereals such as Weetabix, Shredded Wheat, oats and oat bran, unsweetened muesli
● Wholemeal pasta and wholegrain rice
● Peas, beans, lentils in soups or replacing some of the meat in stews
● Vegetables, including potatoes and other roots, salads
● Fruit, fresh, stewed and dried.

Even if you are overweight, foods like potatoes and bread should be part of your diet – they are relatively low in Calories unless you add fat to them. If you are not overweight, it is especially important to eat large portions of these foods to supply the Calories you need whilst reducing the fat in your diet.

These basic foods supply proteins, starch, dietary fibre and many vitamins and minerals.

EAT IN MODERATE

AMOUNTS:

● Lean cuts of red meat, poultry, fish, nuts, eggs:
    Two portions daily of about 4 oz from this list are adequate for most adults. Red meat occasionally will supply iron. Avoid fatty sausages, salami, pates and fatty meats generally.
● The equivalent of half a pint of milk as milk or yoghurt or cheese each day will supply protein, calcium and

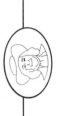

THE QUAKER OATS
NUTRITION CENTRE

important vitamins.
Use skimmed milk, low fat yoghurts and lower fat cheeses like edam or cottage cheese rather than whole milk and dairy products to keep fat intake down.

LIMIT INTAKE OF

THE FOLLOWING:

- Foods high in fat and sugar complete the diet and should be eaten in small amounts.
- Obvious fats include butter, margarines, lard, dripping and oils. Spread butter or margarine thinly on thick slices of bread and avoid adding them to vegetables or use a low fat spread. Avoid fried foods wherever possible.
- Other fatty foods include mayonnaise, salad creams and dressings – look out for lower fat versions if you find salads unpalatable without them.
- Fat is less obvious in foods such as pastry, cakes, sweet, cream or chocolate biscuits, and these foods are high in sugar too. If you aren't overweight, replace these with plain biscuits, crispbreads, muffins or scones.
- Cooking methods are important – grilling, baking, boiling, stewing are better than frying which adds fat. Remove all visible fat from foods and don't fry meat and vegetables for stews and casseroles. If you do fry food, use an oil containing poly-unsaturated fats such as corn, sunflower or safflower oils. Polyunsaturated fats help keep blood cholesterol down.

SUGAR

About half the sugar we eat is added to tea or coffee or cereals or used in cooking at home. The rest comes from sweets, cakes, jams and manufactured foods like soft drinks and fruit flavoured yoghurts.

EAT THE FOLLOWING

ONLY OCCASIONALLY:

- Sugar, sweets, toffees and chocolate, soft drinks and squashes
- Cakes, pastries and sweet biscuits
- Jams, honey, marmalade and syrup
- Sugary puddings including packet mixes, tinned fruit in syrup, ice-cream, jellies
- Sugared breakfast cereals and sweetened muesli
- Sweetened drinks eg drinking chocolate, condensed milk
- Sweet pickles and sauces.

In some cases there are now products available with less sugar, eg canned fruit in natural juice, unsweetened fruit juices, low sugar yoghurts, low calorie squashes and soft drinks. Try these if you still crave something sweet.

SALT IN THE DIET

Keep your salt intake low by adding only small amounts in cooking and not adding salt at table.
Salty foods like bacon, ham, cured meats and fish, cheeses, pickles and sauces are best eaten only two or three times per week at most.

ALCOHOL

The "safe" limit for alcohol intake is said to be 21 units per week for men and 14 for women. It is advisable to keep well below this especially if trying to lose weight since alcohol-containing drinks are high in Calories.
One unit is equal to:

- Half a pint of beer or cider
- One glass of wine
- One small glass of sherry or port
- One measure of spirits.

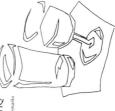

This leaflet is one in a series of five produced by The Quaker Oats Nutrition Centre. If you would like any further information please contact:

The Quaker Oats Nutrition Centre
Dept Q446/Winterhill
Milton Keynes MK6 1HQ

Quaker™ and Quaker Oats™ are trademarks of Quaker Oats Ltd. Year of first publication 1990 Dept Q446/N5.

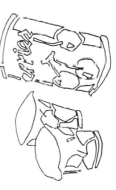

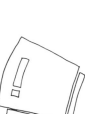

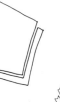

Nutrition Matters

THE HEALTHY WAY

TO LOSE WEIGHT

THE QUAKER OATS
NUTRITION CENTRE

THE HEALTHY WAY TO LOSE

WEIGHT

There is no magic solution to losing weight – it means that you must take in less energy from food than your body requires over a period of time. You need to adjust your eating pattern permanently.
Following the guidelines in this leaflet should help you to lose 1-2lb, on average, each week. This slow and steady loss is much safer than large, rapid weight loss.
Once you have reached your desired weight then you can increase your food intake using these guidelines as a basis. This should mean your new weight will be easier to control.
The guidelines are based around healthy eating principles of:

● More fibre
● Less fat
● Less sugar

BASE YOUR INTAKE AROUND

THESE GROUPS OF FOODS:

MEAT and FISH
Any kind that you like and fits in with your budget. As lean as possible and cooked without the addition of breadcrumbs or fat. Low fat sausages and beefburgers are included, also fishfingers.
CHEESE and EGGS
Look for lower fat cheeses such as Edam, low fat cheddar, low fat cottage and cream cheeses. Do not fry eggs.
MILK and YOGHURT
Use semi-skimmed or skimmed milk only, low fat yoghurts.
FRUIT
Up to four fruits may be taken each day as desired. One fruit is an apple, orange, peach, pear, small banana, a few grapes or strawberries.
VEGETABLES
As many as you like of any sort in order to fill you. Raw or cooked vegetables (no fat added), fresh or frozen. Peas, beans and sweetcorn are particularly good.

EATING

Eat at scheduled times and do nothing else while eating – no watching TV or reading the paper. Store food out of sight. Use a smaller plate. Eat at the table, taking time to relax and enjoy the meal. Don't eat the children's leftovers. Put your knife and fork down between mouthfuls. Chew food thoroughly. Leave food on your plate if you are full. Do not skip meals, especially breakfast.

ON HOLIDAY OR AT SPECIAL OCCASIONS

Enjoy yourself! Plan your day's meals around the special occasion. Eat a low calorie snack before the party. Do not drink too much alcohol – try some low calorie drinks if available.

REMEMBER: A HOLIDAY OR A SPECIAL OCCASION IS TO BE ENJOYED. EATING SOMETHING WHICH IS NOT ON YOUR DIET WILL NOT MAKE ANY DIFFERENCE IN THE LONG TERM.

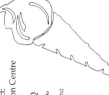

This leaflet is one in a series of five produced by The Quaker Oats Nutrition Centre. If you would like any further information please contact:
The Quaker Oats Nutrition Centre
Dept Q446/Winterhill
Milton Keynes MK6 1HQ

Quaker™ and Quaker Oats™ are trademarks
© Quaker Oats Ltd
Year of first publication 1990. Dept Q446/N2.

TRY TO CUT DOWN ON THE

FOLLOWING GROUPS OF FOODS:

FAT

Use low fat spread. Do not fry – grill, bake or steam instead. Do not eat fatty meat products eg pies, pâtés, pasties, salami, luncheon meat. Remove the skin from poultry. Use low calorie salad dressings. Use low fat milk and cheeses. Avoid snack foods – crisps, nuts and biscuits.

SUGAR

Do not use sugar in tea or coffee, on cereals or fruit, use an artificial sweetener instead. Do not eat chocolate, sweets. Drink low calorie drinks. Avoid sweet puddings – use fruit and yoghurts instead.

REMEMBER: IF YOU DO BREAK YOUR DIET IT'S NOT THE END OF THE WORLD – DON'T GIVE UP – START AFRESH AT THE NEXT MEAL

HINTS TO HELP YOU WHEN:

SHOPPING

Shop for food *after* eating. Don't buy on impulse. Avoid bought made-up dishes unless you know the energy content. Try to plan meals ahead and make a shopping list from your menu.

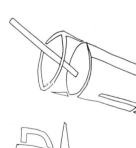

POTATOES, RICE, PULSES, PASTA

Brown rice and pasta are filling, pulses such as lentils are good for extending meat dishes. Potatoes in their jackets (boiled or baked) are good.

BREAD and
BREAKFAST CEREALS

Wholemeal or oat bran bread is best, but all types of bread are really suitable. Up to 5 slices each day should be adequate. Any breakfast cereal which is not sugar-coated is acceptable. A cereal which is high in fibre is even better. Do not add sugar to breakfast cereals.

DRINKS

Tea, coffee, diet fizzy drinks and squashes, mineral water, soda water. Fruit juices contain energy and should be restricted to a small glass with meals. Alcohol should be restricted.

Nutrition Matters

DIETARY ADVICE

TO LOWER BLOOD

CHOLESTEROL

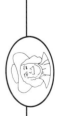

THE QUAKER OATS
NUTRITION CENTRE

TREATMENT OF HIGH

BLOOD LIPIDS

Cholesterol and triglycerides are the two main types of lipids (fats) in the blood. When the levels are high, there may be a high risk of coronary heart disease (CHD). To reduce blood lipids you may need to make these changes to your diet:

● Reduce the energy (calorie) content if you are overweight
● Reduce fat and/or change the type of fat
● Reduce sugar
● Reduce alcohol
● Increase dietary fibre (especially soluble fibre)

But, before making changes, you need to know where you're starting from. Your Practice Nurse will help you to complete the enclosed chart to make a record of your present diet. She may then amend that record to show you how to make any necessary changes in your diet. The following pages set out the general principles of changing diet to lower blood lipids, detailed advice on specific changes will be given by the Practice Nurse.

REDUCING FAT INTAKE

Decreasing the total amount of fat you eat is most important – but replacing some of the saturated fat in the diet with polyunsaturated fats may also help lower your cholesterol level.

So –

Use margarine made from corn, safflower or sunflower oils labelled 'high in Polyunsaturates' to spread on bread. Do not spread thickly.

Use skimmed or semi-skimmed milk instead of whole milk.

Make sure yoghurt is low fat.

Use cottage cheese, curd cheese and low fat hard cheese instead of hard cheeses like cheddar or stilton or cream cheese.

Choose lean cuts of meat and trim off all visible fat before cooking.

Have chicken or turkey or pulses (beans and lentils) at least twice each week.

Eat fish (including fatty fish which is high in polyunsaturates) at least twice each week.

Replace cakes, pastries and pies and sweet biscuits with plain biscuits or crispbreads. Chocolates, toffees and fudge should be a very occasional treat only.

Think about how you cook – grill, bake, braise, boil or steam foods instead of frying.

REDUCING SUGAR INTAKE

If you have a high level of trigly-cerides in your blood or are over-weight then you should cut down on the amount of sugar you eat. Sugar contains only calories and is not a dietary essential.

Try drinking tea and coffee without sugar and do not add it to cereals. If you can't do without the sweet taste use an artificial sweetener eg Sweetex, Canderel or Hermesetas gold.

Use low calorie fizzy drinks and squashes instead of the sweetened versions.

Avoid sweets, peppermints, chocolate and other confectionery and don't regularly eat cakes and sweet biscuits.

LIMIT ALCOHOL INTAKE

Alcohol may raise the level of triglycerides in your blood – it also contains a lot of energy and should be strictly limited if you are trying to lose weight.

Try not to have more than 2-3 drinks three times per week

One drink equals:

- ½ pint beer, cider or lager
- one glass of wine or sherry
- one measure of spirit

Diabetic lagers are high in alcohol and are not recommended

INCREASING DIETARY FIBRE

INTAKE

Increasing intake of starchy foods with a high fibre content helps to replace the calories lost when you cut your fat intake. Some foods high in soluble fibre like oats, oatbran and beans may help lower cholesterol.

Eat wholemeal bread, use wholemeal flour for baking and use wholegrain cereals such as Weetabix and Shredded Wheat. Eat oats, as muesli or porridge, and other oat-based products. Eat wholemeal pasta and brown rice instead of white versions. Eat plenty of fruit and vegetables including potatoes. The skin of vegetables and fruit is high in fibre so eat it when possible. Use pulses like kidney beans, haricot beans, chick peas or lentils to replace some (or all) of the meat in a meal occasionally.

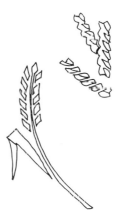

IF YOU NEED TO LOSE

WEIGHT

Limit your intake of margarine to ½ oz per day, or use a low fat spread.
Avoid all fried foods.
Have small portions of meat (3oz) or fish (5oz) for your main meals.
Avoid sweet sugary foods.
Limit bread and potato intake.

This leaflet is one in a series of five produced by The Quaker Oats Nutrition Centre. If you would like any further information please contact:
The Quaker Oats Nutrition Centre
Dept Q446/Winterhill
Milton Keynes MK6 1HQ

Quaker™ and Quaker Oats™ are trademarks of Quaker Oats Ltd
Year of first publication 1990. Dept Q446/N3

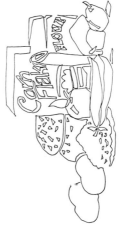

Nutrition Matters

REDUCING
BLOOD PRESSURE

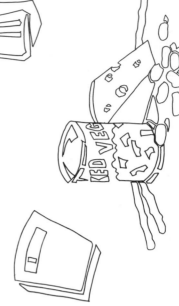

ADVICE TO LOWER BLOOD PRESSURE

High blood pressure or hypertension means blood pressure (BP) which is above the normal level for your age. High blood pressure increases your risk of:

- Heart disease
- Strokes
- Kidney disease

Fortunately there are some steps you can take to reduce these risks.

Consider the following questions:

ARE YOU OVERWEIGHT?

If the answer is yes, simply reducing your weight to a sensible level will help to reduce your BP. A leaflet is available with advice on how to lose weight. If after 4-6 weeks following the advice you haven't lost weight, ask to see a dietitian. If you are at a sensible weight, don't let it go up.

DO YOU EAT TOO MUCH SALT?

Most people in the UK eat more salt than they need and reducing intake can often help reduce BP.

- Do you add a lot of salt when cooking?
- Do you add salt at the table?
- Do you eat salty foods, eg bacon, ham, cheese, smoked or salted fish, more than 3 times per week?
- Do you eat canned meats, fish or vegetables more than once or twice each week?
- Do you eat salted snacks, eg nuts or crisps, every week?

THE QUAKER OATS NUTRITION CENTRE

DO YOU TAKE REGULAR EXERCISE?

Your body needs exercise.
Most physical activity improves circulation and helps to lower BP. Exceptions may be weight-lifting and other very strenuous activities.
Exercise also helps relieve stress. Try going for a walk or swimming two or three times each week. If you haven't done any exercise for a while, start gently and build it up gradually.

DO YOU SMOKE?

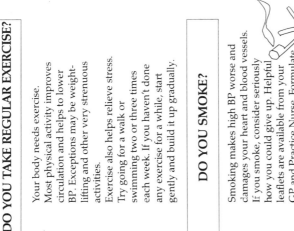

Smoking makes high BP worse and damages your heart and blood vessels.
If you smoke, consider seriously how you could give up. Helpful leaflets are available from your GP and Practice Nurse. Formulate a plan and get those around you to support you in giving up.
HAVE YOUR BLOOD PRESSURE CHECKED REGULARLY ONCE EACH YEAR UNLESS ADVISED TO HAVE IT DONE MORE OFTEN

This leaflet is one in a series of five produced by The Quaker Oats Nutrition Centre. If you would like any further information please contact:
The Quaker Oats Nutrition Centre
Dept Q446/Winterhill
Milton Keynes MK6 1HQ

Quaker™ and Quaker Oats™ are trademarks of Quaker Oats Ltd
Year of first publication 1990. Dept Q446/N1.

DO YOU REGULARLY DRINK

ALCOHOLIC DRINKS?

Too much alcohol can make you fat as well as increase your BP.
The usual upper limits recommended for healthy men (21 units per week) and healthy women (14 units per week) may well be too high for some people with high blood pressure, so you may have to restrict your intake to less than these amounts.
One unit equals:
- Half a pint of beer
- One glass wine
- Single measure of spirits
- Small glass of sherry or port

DO YOU OFTEN FEEL

HARRASSED AND UNDER STRESS?

How to deal with stress:
- Avoid stressful situations
- Don't take on too much
- Take regular exercise
- Stop work and sit and relax at intervals
- If you feel harrassed, stop what you are doing and take some slow, deep breaths
- Talk to someone about the problem

If you answered yes to three or more of these questions, you probably eat too much salt.
To reduce intake:
- Use only a small amount of salt when cooking foods
- Do not add extra salt to the food before eating it

The following foods are high in salt – eat only two or three items per week:
- Table salt, bicarbonate of soda and any foods containing these
- Bacon, ham, gammon, sausages, beefburgers (unless home made), tinned meat, meat pastes and pates
- Smoked or tinned fish eg smoked haddock, cod, mackerel, kippers, fish in brine, fish paste, shell fish
- Cheese especially blue cheese
- Meat or yeast extracts and stock cubes
- Tinned vegetables, baked beans, spaghetti in tomato sauce
- All bottled sauces, ketchup, chutney, salad cream
- Salted savoury or cheese biscuits
- Crisps, salted or roasted peanuts, other savoury snacks

Nutrition Matters

HEALTHY EATING

FOR OLDER PEOPLE

THE QUAKER OATS
NUTRITION CENTRE

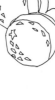

HEALTHY EATING FOR

OLDER PEOPLE

The best way to make sure you get all the nutrients you need is to eat a variety of foods each day. As you get older you may find you want less food than when you were young and if you are eating less food it is important to eat as nourishing a diet as possible.

Choose items from the following groups each day.

Cereals – Bread, breakfast cereals, rice and pasta. Have one (or more) helpings of one of these at each meal eg a bowl of cereal at breakfast, some rice or pasta at midday and two slices of bread as a sandwich in the evening.

Dairy foods – have the equivalent of at least half a pint of milk each day – as milk, yogurt or cheese.

Protein foods – have two portions from this group each day. It includes meat, fish, eggs, beans (eg baked beans, kidney beans, chick peas), nuts, cheese.

Fruit and vegetables – have three to four servings of vegetables (including potatoes and root vegetables) each day. If peeling or chewing fruit is a problem stewed or canned fruit is just as acceptable as fresh.

Make sure you drink enough fluid each day – at least 6 cups of tea, coffee, water or juice.

The above groups are the basis of a good diet – other foods like butter, margarine and oils will add palatability to the diet but if you are overweight it's best to spread them thinly and avoid frying foods. Similarly it's best to use sugar, confectionary, sweet biscuits and pastry as occasional treats if you want to keep your weight down, and not to fill up on these if you have a poor appetite.

As long as your day-to-day diet is good the occasional cream cake, chocolate bar or slap-up meal will do you no harm.

PREPARING MEALS

Shopping may seem a chore, especially if you have transport difficulties but it can be an opportunity to get out of the house and take some exercise. Seeing the range of foods available in the shops may inspire you to try new foods and keep your diet varied.

If you are alone, cooking a meal may seem an effort but it is worth looking after yourself by making sure you get a variety of foods. It doesn't have to be complicated to be nutritious –simple meals like baked beans on toast or cauliflower cheese are inexpensive and easy to prepare. Cooking for other people is often more satisfying –teaming up with a friend or neighbour and cooking for each other can make your diet more interesting and get over the problem of having to buy and cook small quantities.

CONVENIENCE FOODS

There is a wide variety of ready prepared meals and snacks available in the shops now which save the time and effort of cooking – they tend to be more expensive than home made foods but are just as nutritious.

PROBLEMS WITH FOOD

Constipation can be a problem especially if you don't eat much. Don't reach for the laxatives – make sure that you have sufficient dietary fibre by eating wholemeal bread and high-fibre cereals, and make sure you drink enough.

You don't feel like eating – when you aren't feeling well it's difficult to be enthusiastic about eating but if it goes on for more than a few days have a chat with your doctor. Meal replacements can be used and light meals like soups with bread, scrambled eggs, custards or milk puddings or even a bowl of cereal or porridge with milk can help keep you going.

DIFFICULTY PREPARING

FOODS

If you have arthritis or other hand problems it may be difficult to peel and cut foods. New potatoes and carrots and other young vegetables may just need scrubbing rather than peeling and instant potato mashed with butter or margarine is easy to prepare. Remember, too, frozen vegetables are just as nutritious as fresh.

LIVING ON A LIMITED

BUDGET

Food can seem very expensive if you are on a low income especially if you have to buy small quantities of food for one person. Liver, oily fish like herrings or mackerel or sardines, eggs and cheeses are very good value nutritionally and relatively cheap. Look out for fruits and vegetables in season – they are usually cheaper. In the winter thick soups or broth can be made from cheaper cuts of meat or from lentils or beans and vegetables and can be a meal in themselves.

Find out what is available in your area in the way of meals on wheels or luncheon clubs. These often provide a good meal very cheaply.

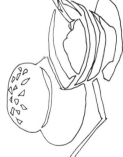

STORE CUPBOARD IDEAS

It's a good idea to keep a small stock of foods for days when the weather is bad or you can't get out to shop. The following would ensure that you could feed yourself well.

UHT milk in cartons.

UHT fruit juices in cartons.

Canned or packet soups.

Canned meat or fish eg corned beef, tuna, sardines, pilchards.

Canned vegetables, instant potatoes, baked beans.

Canned fruits in juice, dried fruit eg prunes, apples, apricots.

Porridge oats and breakfast cereals.

Canned milk puddings.

Crackers and biscuits.

Marmalade, jam, peanut butter, bovril, marmite.

Malted milk, hot chocolate. Complan or Build-Up (meal replacements).

Stock cubes.

'A little of what you fancy does you good!'

This leaflet is one in a series of five produced by The Quaker Oats Nutrition Centre. If you would like any further information please contact:

The Quaker Oats Nutrition Centre

Dept Q446/Winterhill

Milton Keynes MK6 1HQ

Quaker™ and Quaker Oats™ are trademarks of Quaker Oats Ltd. Year of first publication 1990. Dept Q446/N4

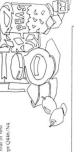

NAME:

FOOD DIARY

HOW TO RECORD YOUR FOOD INTAKE

Please write down everything you eat and drink for five days in the coming week. Make sure that you include at least one weekend day.

Write down the time at the start of each meal or drink or snack. A bar of chocolate eaten at the bus-stop is a snack.

Describe the food as accurately as possible – for instance, a sandwich is actually *three* foods: bread, butter, and eg cheese.

Give clear descriptions of the type of food eaten, eg:

Bread – wholemeal, white, thick or thin sliced

Milk – whole, semi-skimmed, skimmed, evaporated

Sausages – beef or pork, fried or grilled.

Describe the portion in household measures, eg slices, tablespoons, mugs or cups.

EXAMPLE

TIME:	DESCRIPTION OF FOOD OR DRINK:	HOW MUCH:
7.30 am	Boiled egg	1
	White toast	1 slice medium
	Butter (thickly spread)	
	Marmalade	2 teaspoons
	Tea (whole milk, no sugar)	2 cups
9.30 am	Coffee (semi-skimmed milk)	1 cup
	Sugar	1 teaspoon
12.00	Brown bread	1 slice medium
	Cheese	1 oz
	Tomato	1
	Butter (thinly spread)	
	Tea (semi-skimmed milk, no sugar)	1 cup
3.30 pm	Tea (semi-skimmed milk, no sugar)	1 cup
6.00 pm	Beef	2 slices
	Potatoes (new, boiled)	3
	Peas	2 tablespoons
	Gravy	
	Tinned peaches	3 halves
	Ice-cream	1 tablespoon
	Tea (semi-skimmed milk, no sugar)	1 cup

If the spaces in the columns are too small for you, please copy the form onto larger paper.

DAY ONE: DATE:	DAY OF WEEK:		DAY TWO: DATE:	DAY OF WEEK:	
TIME	DESCRIPTION OF FOOD OR DRINK	HOW MUCH	TIME	DESCRIPTION OF FOOD OR DRINK	HOW MUCH

DAY THREE: DATE: DAY OF WEEK:

TIME	DESCRIPTION OF FOOD OR DRINK	HOW MUCH

DAY FOUR: DATE: DAY OF WEEK:

TIME	DESCRIPTION OF FOOD OR DRINK	HOW MUCH

DAY FIVE: DATE: DAY OF WEEK:

TIME	DESCRIPTION OF FOOD OR DRINK	HOW MUCH

Index

Meaning and Medicine

REFLECTIVE BIOETHICS

Series Editors:

Hilde Lindemann Nelson
and James Lindemann Nelson